Basic epidemiology

2nd edition ◄

R Bonita

R Beaglehole

T Kjellström

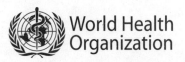 World Health Organization

WHO Library Cataloguing-in-Publication Data

Bonita, Ruth.

   Basic epidemiology / R. Bonita, R. Beaglehole, T. Kjellström. 2nd edition.

   1.Epidemiology. 2.Manuals. I.Beaglehole, Robert. II.Kjellström, Tord. III.World Health Organization.

   ISBN 92 4 154707 3   (NLM classification: WA 105)
   ISBN 978 92 4 154707 9

© World Health Organization 2006

Contents

Preface

Basic epidemiology was originally written with a view to strengthening education, training and research in the field of public health. Since the book was published in 1993, more than 50 000 copies have been printed, and it has been translated into more than 25 languages. A list of these languages and contact addresses of local publishers is available on request from WHO Press, World Health Organization, 1211 Geneva 27, Switzerland.

Basic epidemiology starts with a definition of epidemiology, introduces the history of modern epidemiology, and provides examples of the uses and applications of epidemiology. Measurement of exposure and disease are covered in Chapter 2 and a summary of the different types of study designs and their strengths and limitations is provided in Chapter 3. An introduction to statistical methods in Chapter 4 sets the scene for understanding basic concepts and available tools for analysing data and evaluating the impact of interventions. A fundamental task of epidemiologists is to understand the process of making causal judgements, and this is covered in Chapter 5. The applications of epidemiology to broad areas of public health are covered in the following chapters: chronic noncommunicable disease (Chapter 6), communicable disease (Chapter 7), clinical epidemiology (Chapter 8) and environmental, occupational and injury epidemiology (Chapter 9); the process of health planning is outlined in Chapter 10. The final chapter, Chapter 11, introduces the steps that new epidemiologists can take to further their education and provides links to a number of current courses in epidemiology and public health.

As with the first edition of *Basic epidemiology*, examples are drawn from different countries to illustrate various epidemiological concepts. These are by no means exhaustive or comprehensive and we encourage students and teachers to seek locally relevant examples. Each chapter starts with a few key messages and ends with a series of short questions (answers are provided) to stimulate discussion and review progress.

The authors gratefully acknowledge contributions to the first edition from John Last and Anthony McMichael. Martha Anker wrote Chapter 4 for the first edition. In the second edition, Chapter 4 was written by Professor O. Dale Williams. A version of the course material upon which this chapter is based is available at http://statcourse.dopm.uab.edu.

In addition, the authors would like to thank the following people for their contributions to the second edition: Michael Baker, Diarmid Campbell-Lendrum, Carlos Corvalen, Bob Cummings, Tevfik Dorak, Olivier Dupperex, Fiona Gore, Alec Irwin, Rodney Jackson, Mary Kay Kindhauser, Doris Ma Fat, Colin Mathers, Hoomen Momen, Neal Pearce, Rudolpho Saracci, Abha Saxena, Kate Strong, Kwok-Cho Tang, and Hanna Tolonen. Laragh Gollogly was managing editor, and graphic design was done by Sophie Guetanah-Aguettants and Christophe Grangier.

The International Programme on Chemical Safety (a joint programme of the United Nations Environment Programme, the International Labour Organization, and the World Health Organization), the Swedish International Development Authority (SIDA) and the Swedish Agency for Research Cooperation with Developing Countries (SAREC) all supported the original development of this book.

Introduction

The essential role of epidemiology is to improve the health of populations. This textbook provides an introduction to the basic principles and methods of epidemiology. It is intended for a wide audience, and to be used as training material for professionals in the health and environment fields.

The purpose of this book is to:

- explain the principles of disease causation with particular emphasis on modifiable environmental factors, including environmentally-determined behaviours,
- encourage the application of epidemiology to the prevention of disease and the promotion of health,
- prepare members of the health-related professions for the need for health services to address all aspects of the health of populations, and to ensure that health resources are used to the best possible effect, and
- encourage good clinical practice by introducing the concepts of clinical epidemiology.

At the end of the course the student should be able to demonstrate knowledge of:

- the nature and uses of epidemiology
- the epidemiological approach to defining and measuring the occurrence of health-related states in populations
- the strengths and limitations of epidemiological study designs
- the epidemiological approach to causation
- the contribution of epidemiology to the prevention of disease, the promotion of health and the development of health policy
- the contribution of epidemiology to good clinical practice and
- the role of epidemiology in evaluating the effectiveness and efficiency of health care.

In addition, the student will be expected to have gained a variety of skills, including an ability to:

- describe the common causes of death, disease and disability in her or his community
- outline appropriate study designs to answer specific questions concerning disease causation, natural history, prognosis, prevention, and the evaluation of therapy and other interventions to prevent and control disease.

Chapter 1
What is epidemiology?

Key messages

- Epidemiology is a fundamental science of public health.
- Epidemiology has made major contributions to improving population health.
- Epidemiology is essential to the process of identifying and mapping emerging diseases.
- There is often a frustrating delay between acquiring epidemiological evidence and applying this evidence to health policy.

The historical context

Origins

Epidemiology originates from Hippocrates' observation more than 2000 years ago that environmental factors influence the occurrence of disease. However, it was not until the nineteenth century that the distribution of disease in specific human population groups was measured to any large extent. This work marked not only the formal beginnings of epidemiology but also some of its most spectacular achievements.[1] The finding by John Snow (Box 1.1) that the risk of cholera in London was related to the drinking of water supplied by a particular company provides a well-known example; the map (see Figure 4.1) highlights the clustering of cases. Snow's epidemiological studies were one aspect of a wide-ranging series of investigations that examined related physical, chemical, biological, sociological and political processes.[2]

Comparing rates of disease in subgroups of the human population became common practice in the late nineteenth and early twentieth centuries. This approach was initially applied to the control of communicable diseases (see Chapter 7), but proved to be useful way of linking environmental conditions or agents to specific diseases. In the second half of the twentieth century, these methods were applied to chronic noncommunicable diseases such as heart disease and cancer, especially in middle- and high-income countries.

Recent developments in epidemiology

Epidemiology in its modern form is a relatively new discipline[1] and uses quantitative methods to study diseases in human populations, to inform prevention and control efforts. For example, Richard Doll and Andrew Hill studied the relationship between tobacco use and lung cancer, beginning in the 1950s.[4] Their work was preceded by experimental studies on the carcinogenicity of tobacco tars and by clinical observations linking tobacco use and other possible factors to lung cancer. By using long-term cohort studies, they were able to establish the association between smoking and lung cancer (Figure 1.1).

Box 1.1. Early epidemiological observation

John Snow located the home of each person who died from cholera in London during 1848–49 and 1853–54, and noted an apparent association between the source of drinking-water and the deaths.[3] He compared cholera deaths in districts with different water supplies (Table 1.1) and showed that both the number of deaths and the rate of deaths were higher among people supplied water by the Southwark company. On the basis of his meticulous research, Snow constructed a theory about the communication of infectious diseases and suggested that cholera was spread by contaminated water. He was able to encourage improvements in the water supply long before the discovery of the organism responsible for cholera; his research had a direct and far-reaching impact on public policy.

Snow's work reminds us that public health measures, such as the improvement of water supplies and sanitation, have made enormous contributions to the health of populations, and that in many cases since 1850, epidemiological studies have identified the appropriate measures to take. It is noteworthy, however, that outbreaks of cholera are still frequent among poor populations, especially in developing countries. In 2006, Angola reported 40 000 cholera cases and 1600 deaths; Sudan reported 13 852 cases resulting in 516 deaths in the first few months of the year.

The British doctors cohort has also shown a progressive decrease in death rates among non-smokers over subsequent decades. Male doctors born between 1900–1930 who smoked cigarettes died, on average, about 10 years younger than lifelong non-smokers[5] (Figure 1.2).

Smoking is a particularly clear-cut case, but for most diseases, several factors contribute to causation. Some factors are essential for the development of a disease and some increase the risk of developing disease. New epidemiological methods were needed to analyse these relationships. In low- and middle-income countries where HIV/AIDS, tuberculosis and malaria are common causes of death, communicable disease epidemiology is of vital importance. This branch of epidemiology has now become important in all countries with the emergence of new communicable diseases such as sudden acute respiratory syndrome (SARS), bovine spongiform encephalopathy (BSE), and pandemic influenza. Epidemiology has evolved considerably over the past 50 years and the major challenge now is to explore and act upon the social determinants of health and disease, most of which lie outside the health sector.[6–8]

Table 1.1. Deaths from cholera in districts of London supplied by two water companies,[3] 8 July to 26 August 1854

Water supply company	Population 1851	Cholera deaths (n)	Cholera death rate (per 1000 population)
Southwark	167 654	844	5.0
Lambeth	19 133	18	0.9

Definition, scope, and uses of epidemiology

Definition

Epidemiology as defined by Last[9] is "the study of the distribution and determinants of health-related states or events in specified populations, and the application of this study to the prevention and control of health problems" (see Box 1.2). Epidemiologists are concerned not only with death, illness and disability, but also with more

Figure 1.1. Death rates from lung cancer (per 1000) by number of cigarettes smoked,[4] British male doctors, 1951–1961

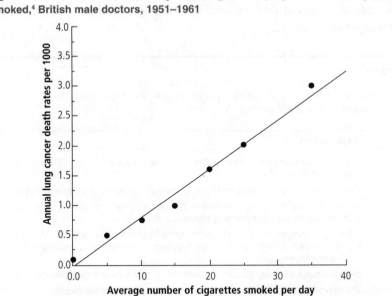

positive health states and, most importantly, with the means to improve health. The term "disease" encompasses all unfavourable health changes, including injuries and mental health.

Scope

A focus of an epidemiological study is the population defined in geographical or other terms; for example, a specific group of hospital patients or factory workers could be the unit of study. A common population used in epidemiology is one selected from a specific area or country at a specific time. This forms the base for defining subgroups

Figure 1.2. Survival from age 35 for continuing cigarette smokers and lifelong non-smokers among British male doctors born 1900–1930 with percentages alive at each decade[5]

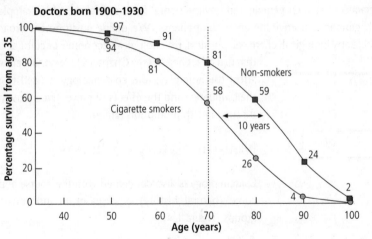

with respect to sex, age group or ethnicity. The structures of populations vary between geographical areas and time periods. Epidemiological analyses must take such variation into account.

Box 1.2. Definition of epidemiology[9]

The word "epidemiology" is derived from the Greek words: *epi* "upon", *demos* "people" and *logos* "study".
   This broad definition of epidemiology can be further elaborated as follows:

Term	Explanation
Study	includes: surveillance, observation, hypothesis testing, analytic research and experiments.
Distribution	refers to analysis of: times, persons, places and classes of people affected.
Determinants	include factors that influence health: biological, chemical, physical, social, cultural, economic, genetic and behavioural.
Health-related states and events	refer to: diseases, causes of death, behaviours such as use of tobacco, positive health states, reactions to preventive regimes and provision and use of health services.
Specified populations	include those with identifiable characteristics, such as occupational groups.
Application to prevention and control	the aims of public health—to promote, protect, and restore health.

Epidemiology and public health

Public health, broadly speaking, refers to collective actions to improve population health.[1] Epidemiology, one of the tools for improving public health, is used in several ways (Figures 1.3–1.6). Early studies in epidemiology were concerned with the causes (etiology) of communicable diseases, and such work continues to be essential since it can lead to the identification of preventive methods. In this sense, epidemiology is a basic medical science with the goal of improving the health of populations, and especially the health of the disadvantaged.

Causation of disease

Although some diseases are caused solely by genetic factors, most result from an interaction between genetic and environmental factors. Diabetes, for example, has both genetic and environmental components. We define environment broadly to include any biological, chemical, physical, psychological, economic or cultural factors that can affect health (see Chapter 9). Personal behaviours affect this interplay, and epidemiology is used to study their influence and the effects of preventive interventions through health promotion (Figure 1.3).

Figure 1.3. Causation

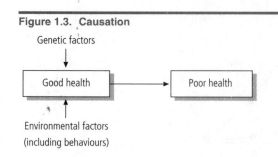

Natural history of disease

Epidemiology is also concerned with the course and outcome (natural history) of diseases in individuals and groups (Figure 1.4).

Figure 1.4. Natural history

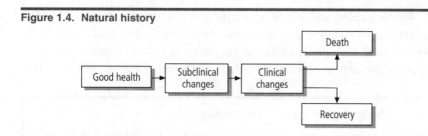

Health status of populations

Epidemiology is often used to describe the health status of population groups (Figure 1.5). Knowledge of the disease burden in populations is essential for health authorities, who seek to use limited resources to the best possible effect by identifying priority health programmes for prevention and care. In some specialist areas, such as environmental and occupational epidemiology, the emphasis is on studies of populations with particular types of environmental exposure.

Figure 1.5. Describing the health status of populations

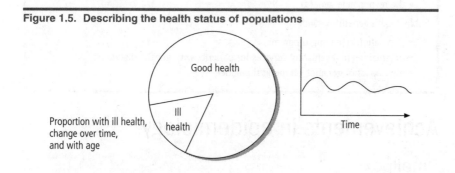

Evaluating interventions

Archie Cochrane convinced epidemiologists to evaluate the effectiveness and efficiency of health services (Figure 1.6).[11] This means determining things such as the appropriate length of stay in hospital for specific conditions, the value of treating high blood pressure, the efficiency of sanitation measures to control diarrhoeal diseases and the impact of reducing lead additives in petrol (see Chapter 10).

Figure 1.6. Evaluating interventions

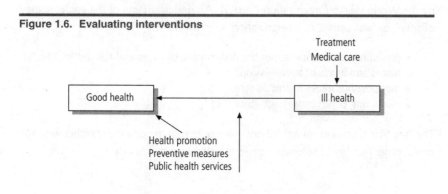

Applying epidemiological principles and methods to problems encountered in the practice of medicine has led to the development of clinical epidemiology (see Chapter 8). Similarly, epidemiology has expanded into other fields such as pharmacoepidemiology, molecular epidemiology, and genetic epidemiology (Box 1.3).[10]

Box 1.3. Molecular and genetic epidemiology

Molecular epidemiology measures exposure to specific substances and early biological response, by:

- evaluating host characteristics mediating response to external agents, and
- using biochemical markers of a specific effect to refine disease categories.

Genetic epidemiology deals with the etiology, distribution, and control of disease in groups of relatives, and with inherited causes of disease in populations.

Genetic epidemiological research in family or population studies aims to establish:

- a genetic component to the disorder,
- the relative size of that genetic effect in relation to other sources of variation in disease risk, and
- the responsible gene(s).

Public health genetics include:

- population screening programs,
- organizing and evaluating services for patients with genetic disorders, and
- the impact of genetics on medical practice.

Achievements in epidemiology

Smallpox

The elimination of smallpox contributed greatly to the health and well-being of millions of people, particularly in many of the poorest populations. Smallpox illustrates both the achievements and frustrations of modern public health. In the 1790s it was shown that cowpox infection conferred protection against the smallpox virus, yet it took almost 200 years for the benefits of this discovery to be accepted and applied throughout the world.

An intensive campaign to eliminate smallpox was coordinated over many years by the World Health Organization (WHO). An understanding of the epidemiology of smallpox was central to its eradication, in particular, by:

- providing information about the distribution of cases and the model, mechanisms and levels of transmission;
- mapping outbreaks of the disease;
- evaluating control measures (Box 1.4).

The fact that there was no animal host was of critical importance together with the low average number of secondary cases infected by a primary case.

When a ten-year eradication programme was proposed by WHO in 1967, 10–15 million new cases and 2 million deaths were occurring annually in 31 countries. The number of countries reporting cases decreased rapidly in the period 1967–76; by 1976 smallpox was reported from only two countries, and the last naturally-occurring case of smallpox was reported in 1977 in a woman who had been exposed to the virus in a laboratory. Smallpox was declared to be eradicated on 8 May 1980.[13]

Several factors contributed to the success of the programme: universal political commitment, a definite goal, a precise timetable, well-trained staff and a flexible strategy. Furthermore, the disease had many features that made its elimination possible and an effective heat-stable vaccine was available. In 1979, WHO maintained a stockpile of smallpox vaccines sufficient to vaccinate 200 million people. This stockpile was subsequently reduced to 2.5 million doses, but given renewed concern about smallpox being used as a biological weapon, WHO continues to maintain and ensure adequate vaccine stocks.[14]

> **Box 1.4. Epidemiological features of smallpox[12]**
>
> Epidemiological methods were used to establish the following features of smallpox:
>
> - there are no non-human hosts,
> - there are no subclinical carriers,
> - recovered patients are immune and cannot transmit the infection,
> - naturally-occurring smallpox does not spread as rapidly as other infectious diseases such as measles or pertussis,
> - transmission is generally via long-lasting human-to-human contact, and
> - most patients are bedridden when they become infectious, which limits transmission.

Methyl mercury poisoning

Mercury was known to be a hazardous substance in the Middle Ages, but has recently become a symbol of the dangers of environmental pollution. In the 1950s, mercury compounds were released with the water discharged from a factory in Minamata, Japan, into a small bay (Box 1.5). This led to the accumulation of methyl mercury in fish, causing severe poisoning in people who ate them.[15]

This was the first known outbreak of methyl mercury poisoning involving fish, and it took several years of research before the exact cause was identified. Minamata disease has become one of the best-documented environmental diseases. A second outbreak occurred in the 1960s in another part of Japan. Less severe poisoning from methyl mercury in fish has since been reported from several other countries.[15, 16]

> **Box 1.5. Minamata disease**
>
> Epidemiology played a crucial role in identifying the cause and in the control of what was one of the first reported epidemics of disease caused by environmental pollution. The first cases were thought to be infectious meningitis. However, it was observed that 121 patients with the disease mostly resided close to Minamata Bay. A survey of affected and unaffected people showed that the victims were almost exclusively members of families whose main occupation was fishing and whose diet consisted mainly of fish. On the other hand, people visiting these families and family members who ate small amounts of fish did not suffer from the disease. It was therefore concluded that something in the fish had caused the poisoning and that the disease was not communicable or genetically determined.[15]

Rheumatic fever and rheumatic heart disease

Rheumatic fever and rheumatic heart disease are associated with poverty, and in particular, with poor housing and overcrowding, both of which favour the spread of streptococcal upper respiratory tract infections. In many affluent countries, the decline in rheumatic fever started at the beginning of the twentieth century, long before the introduction of effective drugs such as sulfonamides and penicillin (Figure 1.7). Today the disease has almost disappeared from most high-income countries although

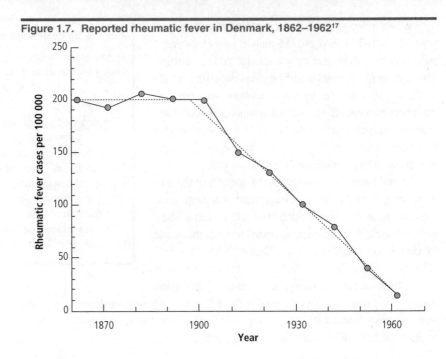

Figure 1.7. Reported rheumatic fever in Denmark, 1862–1962[17]

pockets of relatively high incidence still exist among socially and economically dis-advantaged populations within these countries.

Epidemiological studies have highlighted the role of social and economic factors that contribute to outbreaks of rheumatic fever and to the spread of streptococcal throat infection. Clearly, the causation of these diseases is multifactorial and more complex than that of methyl mercury poisoning, for which there is only one specific causal factor.

Iodine deficiency diseases

Iodine deficiency, which occurs commonly in certain mountainous regions, causes loss of physical and mental energy associated with inadequate production of the iodine-containing thyroid hormone.[18] Goitre and cretinism were first described in detail some 400 years ago, but it was not until the twentieth century that sufficient knowledge was acquired to permit effective prevention and control. In 1915, endemic goitre was named as the easiest known disease to prevent, and use of iodized salt for goitre control was proposed the same year in Switzerland.[18] The first large-scale trials with iodine were done shortly afterwards in Ohio, USA, on 5000 girls aged between 11 and 18 years. The prophylactic and therapeutic effects were impressive and iodized salt was introduced on a community scale in many countries in 1924.

The use of iodized salt is effective because salt is used by all classes of society at roughly the same level throughout the year. Success depends on the effective production and distribution of the salt and requires legislative enforcement, quality control and public awareness (Box 1.6).

Tobacco use, asbestos and lung cancer

Lung cancer used to be rare, but since the 1930s, there has been a dramatic increase in the occurrence of the disease, initially in men. It is now clear that the main cause of increasing lung cancer death rates is tobacco use. The first epidemiological studies linking lung cancer and smoking were published in 1950; five case-control studies reported that tobacco use was associated with lung cancer in men. The strength of the association in the British doctors' study (Figure 1.1) should have been sufficient to evoke a strong and immediate response, particularly as other studies confirmed this association in a wide variety of populations. Had the methods for calculating and interpreting odds ratios been available at the time, the British study referred to in Figure 1.1 would have reported a relative risk of 14 in cigarette smokers compared with never-smokers, too high to be dismissed as bias.[21]

However, other exposures, such as to asbestos dust and urban air pollution also contribute to the increased lung cancer burden. Moreover, the combined effect of smoking and exposure to asbestos is multiplicative, creating exceedingly high lung cancer rates for workers who both smoke and are exposed to asbestos dust (Table 1.2).

Epidemiological studies can provide quantitative measurements of the contribution to disease causation of different environmental factors. Causation is discussed in more detail in Chapter 5.

Table 1.2. Age-standardized lung cancer death rates (per 100 000 population) in relation to tobacco use and occupational exposure to asbestos dust[22]

Exposure to asbestos	History of tobacco use	Lung cancer death rate per 100 000
No	No	11
Yes	No	58
No	Yes	123
Yes	Yes	602

Hip fractures

Epidemiological research on injuries often involves collaboration between scientists in epidemiology and in the social and environmental health fields. Injuries related to falls – particularly fractures of the neck of the femur (hip fractures) in older people – have attracted a great deal of attention in recent years because of the implications for the health service needs of an ageing population. Hip fractures increase exponentially with age as the result of age-related decreased bone mass at the proximal femur and an age-related increase in falls. With the rising number of elderly individuals in most populations, the incidence of hip fracture can be expected to increase proportionately if efforts are not directed towards prevention.

As hip fractures account for a large number of days spent in hospital, the economic costs associated with hip fracture are considerable.[23, 24] In a study of cost of injuries in the Netherlands, hip fracture – which ranked only fourteenth of 25 listed injuries in terms of incidence – was the leading injury diagnosis in terms of costs, accounting for 20% of all costs associated with injury.

Most hip fractures are the result of a fall, and most deaths associated with falls in elderly people result from the complications of hip fractures.[25] The optimal strategies to prevent hip fractures are unclear. Epidemiologists have a vital role in examining both modifiable and non-modifiable factors in an effort to reduce the burden of hip fractures.

HIV/AIDS

The acquired immunodeficiency syndrome (AIDS) was first identified as a distinct disease entity in 1981 in the USA.[26] By 1990, there were an estimated 10 million people infected with the human immunodeficiency virus (HIV). Since then, 25 million people have died of AIDS and a further 40 million have been infected with HIV[27] making it one of the most destructive infectious disease epidemics in recorded history (Figure 1.8).[28]

Figure 1.8. Global AIDS epidemic 1990–2003[28]

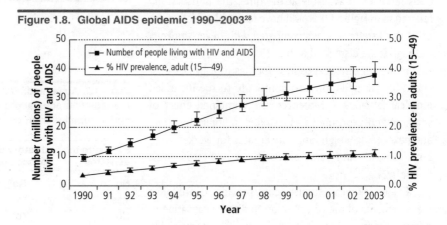

Of the 3.1 million deaths from AIDS in 2005, approximately 95% occurred in low- and middle-income countries, with 70% occurring in sub-Saharan Africa and 20% in Asia.[27] Most of the 4.3–6.6 million people newly infected with HIV in 2005 live in these regions. However, within regions or countries themselves, levels of infection and routes of transmission vary considerably (Box 1.7).

AIDS has a long incubation period and, without treatment, about half of those infected with the causative human immunodeficiency virus (HIV) develop AIDS within nine years of infection (see Chapter 7). The virus is found in blood, semen and cervical or vaginal secretions. Transmission occurs mainly through sexual intercourse or sharing of contaminated needles, but the virus can also be transmitted through transfusion of contaminated blood or blood products, and from an infected woman to her baby during pregnancy, at birth or through breastfeeding.

SARS

Although minor from the perspectives of mortality or burden of disease, the outbreak of sudden acute respiratory syndrome (SARS) reminded the world of the shared vulnerability to new infections.[30, 31] It also highlighted the weakened state of essential public health services, not only in Asia but also in high-income countries such as Canada. SARS first appeared in November 2002 in southern China with two patients with atypical pneumonia of unknown cause. The spread – facilitated by air travel of highly infectious people – was rapid over the following months, causing more than 8000 cases and approximately 900 deaths in 12 countries.[31] Death rates were lower in places where SARS was acquired in the community and higher in hospitals, where health workers had close or repeated contact with infected people.[30]

Box 1.7. HIV, epidemiology, and prevention

Epidemiological and sociological studies have played a vital role in identifying the epidemic, determining the pattern of its spread, identifying risk factors and social determinants, and evaluating interventions for prevention, treatment and control. The screening of donated blood, the promotion of safe sexual practices, the treatment of other sexually transmitted infections, the avoidance of needle-sharing and the prevention of mother-to-child trans-mission with antiretrovirals are the main ways of controlling the spread of HIV/AIDS. With the development of new antiretroviral drugs given in combination, the lives of people with HIV living in high-income countries have been prolonged and improved. The cost of these drugs, however, severely limits their use, and they are currently unavailable to most infected people. A major international effort to scale up treatment of HIV/AIDS – the "3 × 5 cam-paign" (3 million people on treatment by the end of 2005),[29] – managed to get 1 million people on treatment, averting between 250 000 and 350 000 deaths. The next global goal is for universal access to treatment by 2010. Epidemiology has made a major contribution to understanding the AIDS pandemic; however knowledge alone is no guarantee that the appropriate preventive actions will be taken.

Important lessons have been learnt from the experience of responding to the SARS epidemic. For example, SARS has demonstrated that such epidemics can have significant economic and social consequences that go well beyond the impact on health.[32] Such effects show the importance that a severe new disease could assume in a closely interdependent and highly mobile world.[30]

Study questions

1.1   Table 1.1 indicates that there were over 40 times more cholera cases in one district than in another. Did this reflect the risk of catching cholera in each district?

1.2   How could the role of the water supply in causing deaths from cholera have been tested further?

1.3   Why do you suppose the study shown in Figure 1.2 was restricted to doctors?

1.4   What conclusions can be drawn from Figure 1.2?

1.5   Which factors need to be considered when interpreting geographical distri-butions of disease?

1.6   What changes occurred in the reported occurrence of rheumatic fever in Denmark during the period covered in Figure 1.7? What might explain them?

1.7   What does Table 1.2 tell us about the contribution of asbestos exposure and smoking to the risk of lung cancer?

References

1. Beaglehole R, Bonita R. Public health at the crossroads: achievements and prospects. Cambridge, Cambridge University Press, 2004.

2. Johansen PV, Brody H, Rachman S, Rip M. *Cholera, Cholorform, and the Science of Medicine: a life of John Snow.* Oxford, Oxford University Press, 2003

3. Snow J. *On the mode of communication of cholera.* London, Churchill, 1855. (Reprinted in: *Snow on cholera: a reprint of two papers.* New York, Hafner Publishing Company, 1965).

4. Doll R, Hill A. Mortality in relation to smoking: ten years' observations on British doctors. *BMJ* 1964;1:1399-410.

5. Doll R, Peto R, Boreham J, Sutherland I. Mortality in relation to smoking: 50 years' observations on British doctors. *BMJ* 2004;328:1519-28.

6. Lee JW. Public health is a social issue. *Lancet* 2005;365:1005-6.

7. Irwin A, Valentine N, Brown C, Loewenson, R, Solar O, et al. The Commission on Social Determinants of Health: Tackling the social roots of health inequities. *PLoS Med* 2006;3:e106.

8. Marmot M. Social determinants of health inequalities. *Lancet* 2005;365:1099-104.

9. Last JM. *A dictionary of epidemiology,* 4th ed. Oxford, Oxford University Press, 2001.

10. Zimmern RL. Genetics in disease prevention. In: Puncheon D ed, *Oxford Handbook of Public Health Practice.* Oxford, Oxford University Press, 2001:544-549.

11. Cochrane AL. *Effectiveness and Efficiency. Random Reflections on Health Services.* London: Nuffield provincial Provinces Trust, 1972. (Reprinted in 1989 in association with the BMJ; reprinted in 1999 for Nuffield Trust by the Royal Society of Medicine Press, London. ISBN 1-85315-394-X).

12. Moore ZS, Seward JF, Lane M. Smallpox. *Lancet* 2006;367:425-35.

13. Pennington H. Smallpox and bioterrorism. *Bull World Health Organ* 2003;81:762-7.

14. *Global smallpox vaccine reserve: report by the secretariat.* Geneva, World Health Organization, 2004. http://www.who.int/gb/ebwha/pdf_files/EB 115/B115_36_en.pdf

15. McCurry J. Japan remembers Minamata. *Lancet* 2006;367:99-100.

16. *Methylmercury (Environmental health criteria, No 101).* Geneva, World Health Organization, 1990.

17. Taranta A, Markowitz M. *Rheumatic fever: a guide to its recognition, prevention and cure,* 2nd ed. Lancaster, Kluwer Academic Publishers, 1989.

18. Hetzel BS. From Papua to New Guinea to the United Nations: the prevention of mental defect due to iodine deficiency disease. *Aust J Public Health* 1995;19:231-4.

19. De Benoist B, Andersson M, Egli I et al., eds. *Iodine status: worldwide WHO data base on iodine deficiency.* Geneva, World Health Organization, 2004.

20. Hetzel BS. Towards the global elimination of brain damage due to iodine deficiency - the role of the International Council for Control of Iodine Deficiency Disorders. *Int J Epidemiol* 2005;34:762-4.

21. Thun MJ. When truth is unwelcome: the first reports on smoking and lung cancer. *Bull World Health Organ* 2005;83:144-53.

22. Hammond EC, Selikoff IJ, Seidman H. Asbestos exposure, cigarette smoking and death rates. *Ann N Y Acad Sci* 1979;330:473-90.

23. Meerding WJ, Mulder S, van Beeck EF. Incidence and costs of injuries in the Netherlands. *Eur J Public Health* 2006;16:272-78.

24. Johnell O. The socio-economic burden of fractures: today and in the 21st century. [Medline]. *Am J Med* 1997;103:S20-26.

25. Cumming RG, Nevitt MC, Cummings SR. Epidemiology of hip fractures. *Epidemiol Rev* 1997;19:244-57. Medline

26. Gottlieb MS, Schroff R, Schanker HM, Weisman JD, Fan PT, Wolf RA, et al. Pneumocystis carinii pneumonia and mucosal candidiasis in previously healthy homosexual men: evidence of a new acquired cellular immunodeficiency. *N Engl J Med* 1981;305:1425-31.

27. *2004 Report on the global AIDS epidemic: 4th global report.* Geneva, Joint United Nations Programme on HIV/AIDS, 2004

28. *AIDS Epidemic Update: December, 2005.* Geneva, UNAIDS/WHO, 2005.

29. Jong-wook L. Global health improvement and WHO: shaping the future. *Lancet* 2003;362:2083-8.

30. *SARS. How a global epidemic was stopped.* Manila, WHO Regional Office for the Western Pacific, 2006.

31. Wang MD, Jolly AM. Changing virulence of the SARS virus: the epidemiological evidence. *Bull World Health Organ* 2004;82:547-8.

32. *Assessing the impact and costs of SARS in developing Asia. Asian development outlook update 2003.* Asian Development Bank, 2003. http://www.adb.org/Documents/Books/ADO/2003/update/sars.pdf.

Chapter 2
Measuring health and disease

Key messages

- The measure of health and disease is fundamental to the practice of epidemiology.
- A variety of measures are used to characterize the overall health of populations.
- Population health status is not fully measured in many parts of the world, and this lack of information poses a major challenge for epidemiologists.

Defining health and disease

Definitions

The most ambitious definition of health is that proposed by WHO in 1948: *"health is a state of complete physical, mental, and social well-being and not merely the absence of disease or infirmity."*[1] This definition – criticized because of the difficulty in defining and measuring well-being – remains an ideal. The World Health Assembly resolved in 1977 that all people should attain a level of health permitting them to lead socially and economically productive lives by the year 2000. This commitment to the "health-for-all" strategy was renewed in 1998 and again in 2003.[2]

Practical definitions of health and disease are needed in epidemiology, which concentrates on aspects of health that are easily measurable and amenable to improvement.

Definitions of health states used by epidemiologists tend to be simple, for example, "disease present" or "disease absent" (see Box 2.1). The development of criteria to establish the presence of a disease requires a definition of "normality" and "abnormality." However, it may be difficult to define what is normal, and there is often no clear distinction between normal and abnormal, especially with regard to normally distributed continuous variables that may be associated with several diseases (see Chapter 8).

For example, guidelines about cut-off points for treating high blood pressure are arbitrary, as there is a continuous increase in risk of cardiovascular disease at every level (see Chapter 6). A specific cut-off point for an abnormal value is based on an *operational definition* and not on any absolute threshold. Similar considerations apply to criteria for exposure to health hazards: for example, the guideline for a *safe* blood lead level would be based on judgment of the available evidence, which is likely to change over time (see Chapter 9).

Diagnostic criteria

Diagnostic criteria are usually based on symptoms, signs, history and test results. For example, hepatitis can be identified by the presence of antibodies in the blood; asbestosis can be identified by symptoms and signs of specific changes in lung function, radiographic demonstration of fibrosis of the lung tissue or pleural thickening, and a history of exposure to asbestos fibres. Table 2.1 shows that the diagnosis of rheumatic fever diagnosis can be made based on several manifestations of the disease, with some signs being more important than others.

In some situations very simple criteria are justified. For example, the reduction of mortality due to bacterial pneumonia in children in developing countries depends on rapid detection and treatment. WHO's case-management guidelines recommend that pneumonia case detection be based on clinical signs alone, without auscultation, chest radiographs or laboratory tests. The only equipment required is a watch for timing respiratory rate. The use of antibiotics for suspected pneumonia in children–based only on a physical examination – is recommended in settings where there is a high rate of bacterial pneumonia, and where a lack of resources makes it impossible to diagnose other causes.[5]

Likewise, a clinical case definition for AIDS in adults was developed in 1985, for use in settings with limited diagnostic resources.[6] The WHO case definition for AIDS surveillance required only two major signs (weight loss ≥ 10% of body weight, chronic diarrhoea, or prolonged fever) and one minor sign (persistent cough, herpes zoster, generalized lymphadenopathy, etc). In 1993, the Centers for Disease Control defined AIDS to include all HIV-infected individuals with a CD4+ T-lymphocyte count of less than 200 per microlitre.[7]

Box 2.1. Case definition

Whatever the definitions used in epidemiology, it is essential that they be clearly stated, and easy to use and measure in a standard manner in a wide variety of circumstances by different people. A clear and concise definition of what is considered a case ensures that the same entity in different groups or different individuals is being measured.[3] Definitions used in clinical practice are less rigidly specified and often influenced by clinical judgment. This is partly because it is often possible to proceed stepwise with a series of tests until a diagnosis is confirmed.

Table 2.1. Guidelines for the diagnosis of an initial episode of rheumatic fever (Jones criteria, 1992)[4]

A high probability of rheumatic fever is indicated by the presence of two major or one major and two minor manifestations, if supported by evidence of a preceding Group A streptococcal infection[a]

Major manifestations	Minor manifestations
Carditis	**Clinical findings**
Polyarthritis	Arthralgia
Chorea	Fever
Erythema marginatum	**Laboratory findings**
Subcutaneous nodules	Elevated acute-phase reactants:
	— erythrocyte sedimentation rate
	— C-reactive protein
	Prolonged PR interval

[a] Supporting evidence of antecedent Group A streptococcal infection:
— positive throat culture or rapid streptococcal antigen test
— elevated or rising streptococcal antibody titre.

Diagnostic criteria may change quite rapidly as knowledge increases or diagnostic techniques improve; they also often change according to the context in which they are being used. For example, the original WHO diagnostic criteria for myocardial infarction for use in epidemiological studies, were modified when an objective method for assessing electrocardiograms (the Minnesota Code) was introduced in the 1980s.[8, 9] The criteria were further modified in the 1990s, when it became possible to measure cardiac enzymes.[10]

Measuring disease frequency

Several measures of disease frequency are based on the concepts of prevalence and incidence. Unfortunately, epidemiologists have not yet reached complete agreement on the definitions of terms used in this field. In this text we generally use the terms as defined in Last's *Dictionary of Epidemiology.*[11]

Population at risk

An important factor in calculating measures of disease frequency is the correct estimate of the numbers of people under study. Ideally these numbers should only include people who are potentially susceptible to the diseases being studied. For instance, men should not be included when calculating the frequency of cervical cancer (Figure 2.1).

Figure 2.1. Population at risk in a study of carcinoma of the cervix

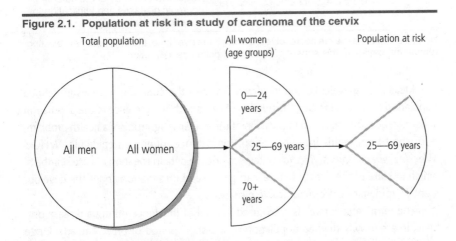

The people who are susceptible to a given disease are called the population at risk, and can be defined by demographic, geographic or environmental factors. For instance, occupational injuries occur only among working people, so the population at risk is the workforce; in some countries brucellosis occurs only among people handling infected animals, so the population at risk consists of those working on farms and in slaughterhouses.

Incidence and prevalence

The incidence of disease represents the rate of occurrence of new cases arising in a given period in a specified population, while prevalence is the frequency of existing cases in a defined population at a given point in time. These are fundamentally different ways of measuring occurrence (see Table 2.2) and the relation between incidence and prevalence varies among diseases. There may be low incidence and a high prevalence – as for diabetes – or a high incidence and a low prevalence – as for the common cold. Colds occur more frequently than diabetes but last only a short time, whereas diabetes is essentially lifelong.

Table 2.2. Differences between incidence and prevalence

	Incidence	Prevalence
Numerator	Number of **new** cases of disease during a specified period of time	Number of **existing** cases of disease at a given point of time
Denominator	Population at risk	Population at risk
Focus	Whether the event is a new case Time of onset of the disease	Presence or absence of a disease Time period is arbitrary; rather a "snapshot" in time
Uses	Expresses the risk of becoming ill The main measure of acute diseases or conditions, but also used for chronic diseases More useful for studies of causation	Estimates the probability of the population being ill at the period of time being studied. Useful in the study of the burden of chronic diseases and implication for health services

Note: If incident cases are not resolved, but continue over time, then they become existing (prevalent) cases. In this sense, prevalence = incidence × duration.

Measuring prevalence and incidence involves the counting of cases in defined populations at risk. Reporting the number of cases without reference to the population at risk can be used to give an impression of the overall magnitude of a health problem, or of short-term trends in a population, for instance, during an epidemic. WHO's *Weekly Epidemiological Record* contains incidence data in the form of case numbers, which in spite of their crude nature, can give useful information about the development of epidemics of communicable diseases.

The term "attack rate" is often used instead of incidence during a disease outbreak in a narrowly-defined population over a short period of time. The attack rate can be calculated as the number of people affected divided by the number exposed. For example, in the case of a foodborne disease outbreak, the attack rate can be calculated for each type of food eaten, and then these rates compared to identify the source of the infection.

Data on prevalence and incidence become much more useful if converted into rates (see Table 1.1). A rate is calculated by dividing the number of cases by the corresponding number of people in the population at risk and is expressed as cases per 10^n people. Some epidemiologists use the term "rate" only for measurements of disease occurrence per time unit (week, year, etc.). In this book, we use the term "disease" in its broad sense, including clinical disease, adverse biochemical and physiological changes, injuries and mental illness.

Prevalence

Prevalence *(P)* of a disease is calculated as follows:

$$P = \frac{\text{Number of people with the disease or condition at a specified time}}{\text{Number of people in the population at risk at the specified time}} (\times 10^{n})$$

Data on the population at risk are not always available and in many studies the total population in the study area is used as an approximation.

Prevalence is often expressed as cases per 100 (percentage), or per 1000 population. In this case, *P* has to be multiplied by the appropriate factor: 10^{n}. If the data have been collected for one point in time, *P* is the "point prevalence rate." It is sometimes more convenient to use the "period prevalence rate," calculated as the total number of cases at any time during a specified period, divided by the population at risk midway through the period. Similarly, a "lifetime prevalence" is the total number of persons known to have had the disease for at least some part of their lives.

Apart from age, several factors determine prevalence (Figure 2.2). In particular:

- the severity of illness (if many people who develop a disease die within a short time, its prevalence is decreased);
- the duration of illness (if a disease lasts a short time its prevalence is lower than if it lasts a long time);
- the number of new cases (if many people develop a disease, its prevalence is higher than if few people do so).

Figure 2.2. Factors influencing prevalence

Increased by:	Decreased by:
Longer duration of the disease	Shorter duration of the disease
Prolongation of life of patients without cure	High case-fatality rate from disease
Increase in new cases (increase in incidence)	Decrease in new cases (decrease in incidence)
In-migration of cases	In-migration of healthy people
Out-migration of healthy people	Out-migration of cases
In-migration of susceptible people	Improved cure rate of cases
Improved diagnostic facilities (better reporting)	

Since prevalence can be influenced by many factors unrelated to the cause of the disease, prevalence studies do not usually provide strong evidence of causality. Measures of prevalence are, however, helpful in assessing the need for preventive action, healthcare and the planning of health services. Prevalence is a useful measure of the occurrence of conditions for which the onset of disease may be gradual, such as maturity-onset diabetes or rheumatoid arthritis.

The prevalence of type 2 diabetes has been measured in various populations using criteria proposed by WHO (see Table 2.3); the wide range shows the importance of social and environmental factors in causing this disease, and indicates the varying need for diabetic health services in different populations.

Table 2.3. Age-adjusted prevalence of type 2 diabetes in selected populations (30–64 years)[12]

Ethnic group population/subgroup		Age-adjusted prevalence (%)	
		Men	Women
Chinese origin			
China		1.6	0.8
Mauritius		16.0	10.3
Singapore		6.9	7.8
Indian origin			
Fiji			
	rural	23.0	16.0
	urban	16.0	20.0
South India			
	rural	3.7	1.7
	urban	11.8	11.2
Singapore		22.7	10.4
Sri Lanka		5.1	2.4

Incidence

Incidence refers to the rate at which new events occur in a population. Incidence takes into account the variable time periods during which individuals are disease-free and thus "at risk" of developing the disease.

In the calculation of incidence, the numerator is the number of new events that occur in a defined time period, and the denominator is the population at risk of experiencing the event during this period. The most accurate way of calculating incidence is to calculate what Last calls the "person-time incidence rate."[11] Each person in the study population contributes one person-year to the denominator for each year (or day, week, month) of observation before disease develops, or the person is lost to follow-up.

Incidence *(I)* is calculated as follows:

$$I = \frac{\text{Number of new events in a specified period}}{\text{Number of persons exposed to risk during this period}} (\times 10^{n})$$

The numerator strictly refers only to first events of disease. The units of incidence rate must always include a unit of time (cases per 10^n and per day, week, month, year, etc.).

For each individual in the population, the time of observation is the period that the person remains disease-free. The denominator used for the calculation of incidence is therefore the sum of all the disease-free person-time periods during the period of observation of the population at risk.

Since it may not be possible to measure disease-free periods precisely, the denominator is often calculated approximately by multiplying the average size of the study population by the length of the study period. This is reasonably accurate if the size of the population is large and stable and incidence is low, for example, for stroke.

In a study in the United States of America, the incidence rate of stroke was measured in 118 539 women who were 30–55 years of age and free from coronary heart disease, stroke and cancer in 1976 (see Table 2.4). A total of 274 stroke cases were identified in eight years of follow-up (908 447 person-years). The overall stroke incidence rate was 30.2 per 100 000 person-years of observation and the rate was higher for smokers than non-smokers; the rate for ex-smokers was intermediate.

Table 2.4. Relationship between cigarette smoking and incidence rate of stroke in a cohort of 118 539 women[13]

Smoking category	Number of cases of stroke	Person-years of observation (over 8 years)	Stroke incidence rate (per 100 000) person-years
Never smoked	70	395 594	17.7
Ex-smoker	65	232 712	27.9
Smoker	139	280 141	49.6
Total	274	908 447	30.2

Cumulative incidence

Cumulative incidence is a simpler measure of the occurrence of a disease or health status. Unlike incidence, it measures the denominator only at the beginning of a study.

The cumulative incidence can be calculated as follows:

$$Cumulative\ Incidence = \frac{\text{Number of people who get a disease during a specified period}}{\text{Number of people free of the disease in the population at risk at the beginning of the period}} (\times 10^n)$$

Cumulative incidence is often presented as cases per 1000 population. Table 2.4 shows that the cumulative incidence for stroke over the eight-year follow-up was 2.3 per 1000 (274 cases of stroke divided by the 118 539 women who entered the study). In a statistical sense, the cumulative incidence is the probability that individuals in the population get the disease during the specified period.

The period can be of any length but is usually several years, or even the whole lifetime. The cumulative incidence rate therefore is similar to the "risk of death" concept used in actuarial and life-table calculations. The simplicity of cumulative incidence rates makes them useful when communicating health information to the general public.

Case fatality

Case fatality is a measure of disease severity and is defined as the proportion of cases with a specified disease or condition who die within a specified time. It is usually expressed as a percentage.

$$Case\ fatality\,(\%) = \frac{\text{Number of deaths from diagnosed cases in a given period}}{\text{Number of diagnosed cases of the disease in the same period}} \times 100$$

Interrelationships of the different measures

Prevalence is dependent on both incidence and disease duration. Provided that the prevalence *(P)* is low and does not vary significantly with time, it can be calculated approximately as:

$$P = \text{incidence} \times \text{average duration of disease}$$

The cumulative incidence rate of a disease depends on both the incidence and the length of the period of measurement. Since incidence usually changes with age, age-specific incidence rates need to be calculated. The cumulative incidence rate is a useful approximation of incidence when the rate is low or when the study period is short.

Figure 2.3 illustrates the various measures of disease. This hypothetical example is based on a study of seven people over seven years.

Figure 2.3. Calculation of disease occurrence

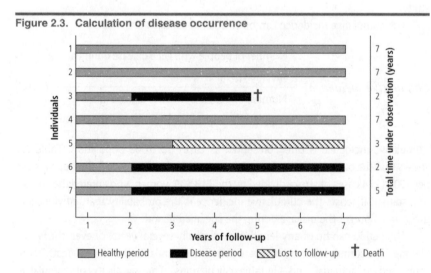

In Figure 2.3 it can be seen that:

- **the incidence** of the disease during the seven-year period is the number of new events (3) divided by the sum of the lengths of time at risk of getting the disease for the population (33 person-years), i.e. 9.1 cases per 100 person-years;

- **the cumulative incidence** is the number of new events in the population at risk (3) divided by the number of people in the same population free of the disease at the beginning of the period (7), i.e. 43 cases per 100 persons during the seven years;
- **the average duration** of disease is the total number of years of disease divided by the number of cases, i.e. 13/3 = 4.3 years;
- **the prevalence** depends on the point in time at which the study takes place; at the start of year 4, for example, it is the ratio of the number of people with the disease (2) to the number of people in the population observed at that time (6), i.e. 33 cases per 100 persons. The formula given on page for prevalence would give an estimated average prevalence of 30 cases per 100 population (9.1 × 3.3);
- **case fatality** is 33% representing 1 death out of 3 diagnosed cases.

Using available information to measure health and disease

Mortality

Epidemiologists often investigate the health status of a population by starting with information that is routinely collected. In many high-income countries the fact and cause of death are recorded on a standard death certificate, which also carries information on age, sex, and place of residence. The *International Statistical Classification of Diseases and Related Health Problems* (ICD) provides guidelines on classifying deaths.[14] The procedures are revised periodically to account for new diseases and changes in case-definitions, and are used for coding causes of death (see Box 2.2). The International Classification of Diseases is now in its 10th revision, so it is called the ICD-10.

Box 2.2. International Classification of Diseases (ICD)

The ICD-10 came into use in 1992. This classification is the latest in a series which originated in the 1850s. The ICD has become the standard diagnostic classification for all general epidemiological and many health management purposes.

The ICD-10 is used to classify diseases and other health problems recorded on many types of records, including death certificates and hospital charts. This classification makes it possible for countries to store and retrieve diagnostic information for clinical and epidemiological purposes, and compile comparable national mortality and morbidity statistics.

Limitations of death certificates

Data derived from death statistics are prone to various sources of error but, from an epidemiological perspective, often provide invaluable information on trends in a population's health status. The usefulness of the data depends on many factors, including the completeness of records and the accuracy in assigning the underlying causes of death—especially in elderly people for whom autopsy rates are often low.

Epidemiologists rely heavily on death statistics for assessing the burden of disease, as well as for tracking changes in diseases over time. However, in many countries basic mortality statistics are not available, usually because of a lack of resources to establish routine vital registration systems. The provision of accurate cause-of-death information is a priority for health services.[15]

Limitations of vital registration systems

The WHO Mortality Database includes only one third of adult deaths in the world, and these are mainly in high-income and middle-income countries.[16, 17] Not all countries are able to submit mortality data to WHO, and for some there are concerns about the accuracy of the data. In some countries, the vital registration system covers only part of the country (urban areas, or only some provinces). In other countries, although the vital registration system covers the whole country, not all deaths are registered. Some countries rely on validation of deaths from representative samples of the population (as in China and India); in other countries, demographic surveillance sites provide mortality rates for selected populations.[18]

Verbal autopsy

A verbal autopsy is an indirect method of ascertaining biomedical causes of death from information on symptoms, signs and circumstances preceding death, obtained from the deceased person's family.[19] In many middle- and low-income countries, verbal autopsy is the only method used to obtain estimates of the distribution of the causes of death.[20] Verbal autopsies are used mainly in the context of demographic surveillance and sample registration systems. The diversity of tools and methods used makes it difficult to compare cause-of-death data between places over time.[21]

Towards comparable estimates

Even in countries where underlying causes of death are assigned by qualified staff, miscoding can occur. The main reasons for this are:

- systematic biases in diagnosis
- incorrect or incomplete death certificates
- misinterpretation of ICD rules for selection of the underlying cause
- variations in the use of coding categories for unknown and ill-defined causes.

For these reasons, data comparisons between countries can be misleading. WHO works with countries to produce country-level estimates, which are then adjusted to account for these differences (see Box 2.3).

Box 2.3. Comparable estimates derived from official statistics

An assessment of the global status of cause of death data suggests that of the 192 Member States of WHO, only 23 countries have high-quality data defined as:

- data are more than 90% complete
- ill-defined causes of death account for less than 10% of the total causes of death
- ICD-9 or ICD-10 codes are used.

The country-level estimates that WHO produces adjust for differences in completeness and accuracy of data supplied by countries. Estimates are based on data from 112 national vital registration systems that capture about 18.6 million deaths annually, representing one third of all deaths occurring in the world. Information from sample registration systems, population laboratories and epidemiological studies are also used to improve these estimates.

Where national vital registration systems do exist and are included in the WHO Mortality Database:

- death certificates may not be complete
- poorer segments of populations may not be covered
- deaths may not be reported for cultural or religious reasons
- the age at death may not be given accurately.

Other factors contributing to unreliable registration systems include: late registration, missing data and errors in reporting or classifying the cause of death.[19]

As it takes a long time for countries to build good quality vital registration systems, alternative methods are often used to assign cause-of-death and to estimate mortality.

Death rates

The death rate (or crude mortality rate) for all deaths or a specific cause of death is calculated as follows:

$$Crude\ mortality\ rate = \frac{\text{Number of deaths during a specified period}}{\text{Number of persons at risk of dying during the same period}}\ (\times 10^n)$$

The main disadvantage of the crude mortality rate is that it does not take into account the fact that the chance of dying varies according to age, sex, race, socio-economic class and other factors. It is not usually appropriate to use it for comparing different time periods or geographical areas. For example, patterns of death in newly occupied urban developments with many young families are likely to be very different from those in seaside resorts, where retired people may choose to live. Comparisons of mortality rates between groups of diverse age structure are usually based on age-standardized rates.

Age-specific death rates

Death rates can be expressed for specific groups in a population which are defined by age, race, sex, occupation or geographical location, or for specific causes of death. For example, an age- and sex-specific death rate is defined as:

$$\frac{\begin{array}{l}\text{Total number of deaths occurring in a specific age and sex group}\\ \text{of the population in a defined area during a specified period}\end{array}}{\begin{array}{l}\text{Estimated total population of the same age and sex group of the}\\ \text{population in the same area during the same period}\end{array}}(\times 10^n)$$

Proportionate mortality

Occasionally the mortality in a population is described by using proportionate mortality, which is actually a ratio: the number of deaths from a given cause per 100 or 1000 total deaths in the same period. Proportionate mortality does not express the risk of members of a population contracting or dying from a disease.

Comparisons of proportionate rates between groups may show interesting differences. However, unless the crude or age-group-specific mortality rates are known, it may not be clear whether a difference between groups relates to variations in the numerators or the denominators. For example, proportionate mortality rates for cancer would be much greater in high-income countries with many old people than in low- and middle-income countries with few old people, even if the actual lifetime risk of cancer is the same.

Infant mortality

The infant mortality rate is commonly used as an indicator of the level of health in a community. It measures the rate of death in children during the first year of life, the denominator being the number of live births in the same year.

The infant mortality rate is calculated as follows:

$$\textit{Infant mortality rate} = \frac{\text{Number of deaths in a year of children less than 1 year of age}}{\text{Number of live births in the same year}} \times 1000$$

The use of infant mortality rates as a measure of overall health status for a given population is based on the assumption that it is particularly sensitive to socioeconomic changes and to health care interventions. Infant mortality has declined in all regions of the world, but wide differences persist between and within countries (see Figure 2.4).

Figure 2.4. Worldwide trends in infant mortality, 1950–2000[22]

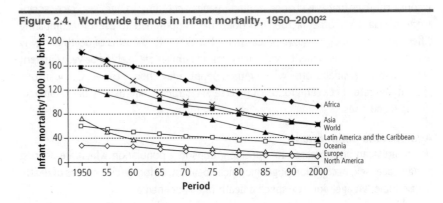

Child mortality rate

The child mortality rate (under-5 mortality rate) is based on deaths of children aged 1–4 years, and is frequently used as a basic health indicator. Injuries, malnutrition and infectious diseases are common causes of death in this age group. The under-5 mortality rate describes the probability (expressed per 1000 live births) of a child dying before reaching 5 years of age. Table 2.5 shows the mortality rates for countries representing a range of income categories. The areas of uncertainty around the estimates for middle-income and low-income countries are shown in parentheses.

Data in Table 2.5 have been calculated so that the information can be compared between countries. Mortality rates per 1000 live births vary from as low as 4 for Japan (based on precise data) to 297 for males in Sierra Leone (with a wide range of uncertainty: between 250 and 340 per 1000 live births).[23] Gathering accurate data is not easy and alternative approaches have been developed (see Box 2.4).

Table 2.5. Under-5 mortality rates in selected countries, 2003[23]

Country	Under-5 mortality rate per 1000 live births (95% CI)	
	Males	**Females**
High-income countries		
Japan	4	4
France	5	5
Canada	6	5
USA	9	7
Middle-income countries		
Chile	10 (9–11)	9 (8–10)
Argentina	19 (18–21)	16 (15–17)
Peru	36 (31–42)	32 (27–39)
Indonesia	45 (40–49)	37 (33–40)
Low-income countries		
Cuba	8 (7–10)	6 (5–7)
Sri Lanka	17 (14–19)	13 (11–15)
Angola	276 (245–306)	243 (216–276)
Sierra Leone	297 (250–340)	270 (229–310)

Box 2.4. Alternative approaches to obtaining information on deaths in children

Where accurate death registers do not exist, infant and child mortality can be estimated from information collected in household surveys in which the following question is initially asked: "During the last two years, have any children in this household died who were aged five years or less?"

If the answer is "yes," three questions are asked:

- "How many months ago did the death occur?"
- "How many months of age was the child at death?"
- "Was the child a boy or a girl?"

If information on the number and ages of surviving children is collected during a survey, infant and child mortality rates can be estimated with reasonable accuracy. Adult mortality can also be approximated from household surveys if accurate information is not available.

Problems with using household surveys to obtain information on deaths include:

- respondents may not understand the time span of the question,
- children who die shortly after birth may be left out,
- for cultural reasons, more male than female deaths may be reported.

However, this is the only method that is applicable in some communities. Measurement of infant mortality in low-income communities is particularly important in helping planners to address the need for equity in health care. Additionally, reducing child mortality rates is one of the Millennium Development Goals (see Chapter 10).

Maternal mortality rate

The maternal mortality rate refers to the risk of mothers dying from causes associated with delivering babies, complications of pregnancy or childbirth. This important statistic is often neglected because it is difficult to calculate accurately. The maternal mortality rate is given by:

$$Maternal\ mortality\ rate = \frac{\begin{array}{c}\text{Number of maternal deaths from} \\ \text{puerperal causes in a given geographic} \\ \text{area in a given year}\end{array}}{\begin{array}{c}\text{Number of live births that occurred} \\ \text{among the population of the given} \\ \text{geographic area during the same year}\end{array}}(\times 10^7)$$

The maternal mortality rate ranges from about 3 per 100 000 live births in high-income countries to over 1500 per 100 000 live births in low-income countries.[23] However, even this comparison does not adequately reflect the much greater lifetime risk of dying from pregnancy-related causes in poorer countries.

Adult mortality rate

The adult mortality rate is defined as the probability of dying between the ages of 15 and 60 years per 1000 population. The adult mortality rate offers a way to analyse health gaps between countries in the main working age groups.[24] The probability of dying in adulthood is greater for men than for women in almost all countries, but the variation between countries is very large. In Japan, less than 1 in 10 men (and 1 in 20 women) die in these productive age groups, compared with almost 2 in 3 men (and 1 in 2 women) in Angola (see Table 2.6).

Table 2.6. Adult mortality rates[25] in selected countries, 2004

Country	Probability of dying per 1000 population between 15 and 60 years	
	Males	**Females**
High-income countries		
Japan	92	45
Canada	91	57
France	132	60
USA	137	81
Middle-income countries		
Chile	133	66
Argentina	173	90
Peru	184	134
Indonesia	239	200
Low-income countries		
Cuba	131	85
Sri Lanka	232	119
Angola	591	504
Sierra Leone	579	497

Life expectancy

Life expectancy is another summary measure of the health status of a population. It is defined as the average number of years an individual of a given age is expected to live if current mortality rates continue. It is not always easy to interpret the reasons for the differences in life expectancy between countries; different patterns may emerge according to the measures that are used.

For the world as a whole, life expectancy at birth has increased from 46.5 years during the period 1950–1955 to 65.0 years during the period 1995–2000 (see Figure 2.5). Reversals in life expectancy have occurred in some sub-Saharan countries largely due to AIDS. Similar reversals in life expectancy have also occurred in middle-aged men in the former Soviet Union, where almost 1 in 2 men die between the ages of 15 and 60 years, largely due to changes in the use of alcohol and tobacco.[26]

Life expectancy at birth, as an overall measure of health status, attaches greater importance to deaths in infancy than to deaths later in life. Table 2.7 gives data

Figure 2.5. Worldwide trends in life expectancy, 1950–2000[28]

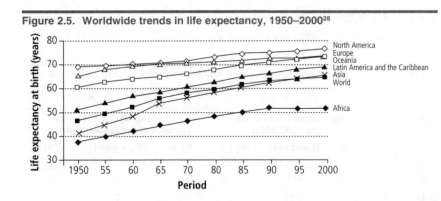

for selected countries. As the data are based on existing age-specific death rates, additional calculation is necessary to allow comparability between countries; the uncertainty of the estimates are shown in parentheses. Confidence intervals can be quite large – as in Zimbabwe – but quite precise in countries like Japan which has complete vital registration.

These data show the large variations in life expectancies between countries. For example, a girl born in Japan in 2004 can expect to live 86 years, whereas a girl born in Zimbabwe at the same time will live between 30 and 38 years. In almost all countries, women live longer than men.[27]

Table 2.7. Life expectancy at birth for men and women in selected countries[28]

Country	Life expectancy at birth (years)	
	Women	Men
Zimbabwe	34 (30–38)	37 (34–40)
Russian Federation	72	59
Egypt	70	66
China	74	70
Mexico	77	72
USA	80	75
Japan	86	79

Age-standardized rates

An age-standardized death rate (also referred to as an age-adjusted rate) is a summary measure of the death rate that a population would have if it had a standard age structure. The standardization of rates can be done either directly or indirectly (see Box 2.5).

Age-standardized rates enable comparisons to be made between populations that have different age structures. Standardization can also be done for variables other than age. This is necessary when comparing two or more populations that have different basic characteristics that independently influence the risk of death (such as age, race, socioeconomic status, etc.).

Frequently used standard populations include:

- the Segi world population[29]
- the European standard population based on the Swedish population
- the WHO world standard population, which is based on world overall average projected populations 2000–2025.[30]

Box 2.5. Direct and indirect standardization of disease rates

The direct method of standardization is more frequently used, and is done by applying the disease rates of the populations being compared to a standard population. This method yields the number of cases that would be expected if the age-specific rates in the standard population were true for the study population.

Standardized rates are used, whenever relevant, for morbidity as well as mortality. The choice of a standard population is arbitrary, but can be problematic when comparing rates of low-income and high-income countries.

Details on methods of standardizing rates can be found in: *Teaching health statistics: lesson and seminar outlines.*[31]

While each give different age-standardized rates (see Table 2.8), they generally do not affect the overall ranking when comparing rates of different populations.[30]

Table 2.8. Directly standardized male death rates from respiratory infections, and the ranking of five countries using three different standard populations[30]

Country	Age-standardized rate (per 100 000)			Ranking of countries by age-standardized rate		
	Segi	European	WHO world	Segi	European	WHO world
Australia	6.3	10.1	7.9	5	5	5
Cuba	27.2	44.2	34.6	4	4	4
Mauritius	45.2	72.6	56.6	3	3	3
Singapore	71.9	120.8	93.3	2	1	1
Turkmenistan	114.2	87.9	91.2	1	2	2

The age-standardization of rates eliminates the influence of different age distributions on the morbidity or mortality rates being compared. For example, there is great variation between countries in the reported crude mortality rates for heart disease as shown in Table 2.9. Finland has a crude heart disease death rate approximately three times that of Brazil, but the standardized rate is the same. Similarly, the United States of America has a crude rate more than twice that of Brazil, yet again, age-standardized rates are similar. Thus the difference between these countries is not as large as it appears from the crude rates.

High-income countries have a much greater proportion of older people in their populations than low- and middle-income countries—the older people have higher rates of cardiovascular disease compared with younger people. All these death rates are influenced by the quality of the original data on the causes of death.

Table 2.9. Crude and age-standardized death rates (per 100 000) for heart disease in three selected countries (men and women combined), 2002

Country	Crude death rate	Age-standardized death rate
Brazil	79	118
Finland	240	120
USA	176	105

Morbidity

Death rates are particularly useful for investigating diseases with a high case-fatality. However, many diseases have low case-fatality, for example, most mental illnesses, musculoskeletal diseases, rheumatoid arthritis, chickenpox and mumps. In this situation, data on morbidity (illness) are more useful than mortality rates.

Morbidity data are often helpful in clarifying the reasons for particular trends in mortality. Changes in death rates could be due to changes in morbidity rates or in case-fatality. For example, the recent decline in cardiovascular disease mortality rates in many developed countries could be due to a fall in either incidence (suggesting improvements in primary prevention) or in case-fatality (suggesting improvements in treatment). Because population age structures change with time, time-trend analyses should be based on age-standardized morbidity and mortality rates.

Other sources of morbidity data include:

- hospital admissions and discharges
- outpatient and primary health care consultations
- specialist services (such as injury treatment)
- registers of disease events (such as cancer and congenital malformations).

To be useful for epidemiological studies, the data must be relevant and easily accessible. In some countries, the confidential nature of patient medical records may make hospital data inaccessible for epidemiological studies. A recording system focusing on administrative or financial data, rather than on diagnostic and individual characteristics may diminish the epidemiological value of routine health service data. Hospital admission rates are influenced by factors other than the morbidity of the population, such as the availability of beds, hospital admission policies and social factors.

Because of the numerous limitations of routinely recorded morbidity data, many epidemiological studies of morbidity rely on the collection of new data using specially designed questionnaires and screening methods. This enables investigators to have more confidence in the data and the rates calculated from them.

Disability

Epidemiologists are concerned not only the occurrence of disease, but also the consequences of disease: impairments, disabilities and handicaps. These have been defined by the WHO International Classification of Functioning, Disability and Health (ICF).[32]

ICF describes how people live with their health condition. The domains are classified from body, individual and societal perspectives. Since an individual's functioning and disability occurs within a context, ICF also includes a list of environmental factors. ICF is a useful tool for understanding and measuring health outcomes. It can be used in clinical settings, health services or surveys, at the individual or population level.

The key parameters of ICF are as follows:

- **impairment**: any loss or abnormality of psychological, physiological or anatomical structure or function;
- **disability**: any restriction or lack (resulting from an impairment) of ability to perform an activity in the manner or within the range considered normal for a human being;
- **handicap**: a disadvantage for a given individual, resulting from an impairment or a disability, that limits or prevents the fulfilment of a role that is normal (depending on age, sex, and social and cultural factors) for that individual.

The relationship between the different non-fatal outcomes is shown in Box 2.6.

Box 2.6. Schema for assessing non-fatal health outcomes

Disease	→	Impairment	→	Disability	→	Handicap
Polio		Paralyzed legs		Inability to walk		Unemployed
Brain injury		Mild mental retardation		Difficulty in learning		Social isolation

It is difficult to measure the prevalence of disability, but it is becoming increasingly important in societies where acute morbidity and fatal illness are decreasing, and where there is an increasing number of aged people living with disabilities.

Health determinants, indicators, and risk factors

Health determinants

Health determinants are generally defined as the underlying social, economic, cultural and environmental factors that are responsible for health and disease, most of which are outside the health sector.[33–35]

Health indicators

A health indicator is a variable – that can be measured directly to reflect the state of health of people within a community. WHO presents the most recent data for 50 health indicators each year.[25] Health indicators can also be used as components in the calculation of a broader social development index. The best example is the Human Development Index, which ranks countries each year according to a combination of the level of economic development, literacy, education, and life expectancy (http://hdr.undp.org/).

Risk factors

A risk factor refers to an aspect of personal habits or an environmental exposure, that is associated with an increased probability of occurrence of a disease. Since risk factors can usually be modified, intervening to alter them in a favourable direction can reduce the probability of occurrence of disease. The impact of these interventions can be determined by repeated measures using the same methods and definitions (see Box 2.7).

Box 2.7. Measuring risk factors

Risk factors can include tobacco and alcohol use, diet, physical activity, blood pressure and obesity. Since risk factors can be used to predict future disease, their measurement at a population level is important, but also challenging.

Tobacco use can be measured by self-reported exposure (yes/no), quantity of cigarettes smoked, or by biological markers (serum cotinine). However, different surveys use different methods, often with different measurement techniques and criteria for detecting a risk factor or clinical outcome (for example, diabetes or hypertension). Additionally, surveys may only be representative of small population groups within a country, district or city. These methodological differences mean that it is be difficult to compare results from different surveys and countries.

Efforts have been made to standardize methods of measurement of risk factors at the global level, including the WHO MONICA Project in the 1980s and 1990s.[36, 37] More recently, the WHO STEPS approach to the measurement of population levels of risk factors provides methods and materials to encourage countries to collect data in a standardized manner.[38, 39]

Data from individual countries can be adjusted to account for known biases to make them internationally comparable. This step is also necessary because countries conduct standard surveys at different times. If risk factor rates are changing over time, information on trends will be needed to adjust data to a standard reporting year.

Other summary measures of population health

Policy-makers face the challenge of responding to current disease prevention and control priorities, while being responsible for predicting future priorities. Such decisions should be based on summary measures that quantify the amount of disease at the population level. These measures need to combine deaths and time spent in ill-health in an internally consistent way, using a common unit of measurement.

Such summary measures serve as a common currency for reporting the burden of disease in populations. They provide a way of monitoring and evaluating population health, so that prevention and control actions can be taken rapidly when necessary.

Mortality alone does not provide a full picture of how different causes affect population health. Duration of life combined with some notion of its quality are reflected in the following population measures:

- years of potential life lost (PLL) based on the years of life lost through premature death (before an arbitrarily determined age);
- healthy life expectancy (HALE);
- disability-free life expectancy (DFLE);
- quality-adjusted life years (QALYs);
- disability-adjusted life years (DALYs).

Disability-adjusted life years

The Global Burden of Disease project[40] combines the impact of premature mortality with that of disability. It captures the population impact of important fatal and non-fatal disabling conditions through a single measure. The major measure used is disability-adjusted life years (DALYs) which combines:

- years of lost life (YLL) – calculated from the number of deaths at each age multiplied by a global standard life expectancy for the age at which death occurs
- years lost to disability (YLD), where the number of incident cases due to injury and illness is multiplied by the average duration of the disease and a weighting factor reflecting the severity of the disease on a scale from 0 (perfect health) to 1 (dead).

One DALY is one lost year of "healthy" life and the measured disease burden is the gap between a population's current health status and that of an ideal situation where everyone lives into old age, free of disability. The normative reference population has a life expectancy at birth of 82.5 years for females and 80.0 years for males.[40]

Time-discounting and non-uniform age weights, which give less weight to years lived at young and older ages, are used in calculating standard DALYs as reported in recent WHO World Health Reports. With age weights and time discounting, a death in infancy corresponds to 33 DALYs, and deaths from ages 5 to 20 to around 36 DALYs. Thus a disease burden of 3300 DALYs in a population would be the equivalent of 100 infant deaths or to approximately 5500 persons aged 50 years living one year with blindness (disability weighting = 0.6).

DALYs were designed to guide World Bank investment policies for health and to inform global priority setting for health research and international health programs.[41] Analysis of DALYs due to a variety of causes and risk factors has given new perspectives on the relative importance of different areas of disease prevention.[42]

Comparing disease occurrence

Measuring the occurrence of disease or other health states is the first step of the epidemiological process. The next step is comparing occurrence in two or more groups of people whose exposures have differed. An individual can be either exposed or unexposed to a factor under study. An unexposed group is often used as a reference group. Exposed people can have different levels and durations of exposure (see Chapter 9). The total amount of a factor that reaches an individual is called the "dose."

We can then compare occurrences to calculate the risk that a health effect will result from an exposure. We can make both absolute and relative comparisons; the measures describe the strength of an association between exposure and outcome.

Absolute comparisons

Risk difference
The risk difference, also called excess risk, is the difference in rates of occurrence between exposed and unexposed groups in the population. It is a useful measure of the extent of the public health problem caused by the exposure. For example, from the data in Table 2.4 the risk difference between the incidence rate of stroke in women who smoke, and the rate of stroke in women who have never smoked, is 31.9 per 100 000 person-years.

When comparing two or more groups, it is important that they are as similar as possible, with the exception of the factor being analysed. If the groups differ in relation to age, sex, etc. the rates must be standardized before a comparison can be made.

Attributable fraction (exposed)
The attributable fraction (exposed), also known as the etiological fraction (exposed), is the proportion of all cases that can be attributed to a particular exposure. We can determine the attributable fraction (AF) by dividing the risk (or attributable) difference by the incidence among the exposed population. For the data in Table 2.4 the attributable fraction of smoking for stroke in the smokers is: $((49.6 - 17.7)/49.6) \times 100 = 64\%$.

When a particular exposure is believed to be a cause of a given disease, the attributable fraction is the proportion of the disease in the specific population that would be eliminated if the exposure were eliminated. In the above example, one would expect to achieve a 64% reduction in the risk of stroke among the women smokers if smoking were stopped, based on the assumption that smoking is both causal and preventable.

Attributable fractions are useful for assessing priorities for public health action. For example, both smoking and air pollution are causes of lung cancer, but the attributable fraction due to smoking is usually much greater than that due to air pollution. Only in communities with very low smoking prevalence and severe air pollution is the latter likely to be the major cause of lung cancer. In most countries, smoking control should take priority in lung cancer prevention programmes.

Population attributable risk

The population attributable risk (*PAR*) is the incidence of a disease in a population that is associated with (or attributed to) an exposure to a risk factor.[11] This measure is useful for determining the relative importance of exposures for the entire population. It is the proportion by which the incidence rate of the outcome in the entire population would be reduced if exposure were eliminated.

PAR can be estimated by the formula:

$$PAR = \frac{I_p - I_u}{I_p}$$

where

I_p is the incidence of the disease in the total population and

I_u is the incidence of the disease among the unexposed group.

Relative comparisons

Relative risk

The relative risk (also called the risk ratio) is the ratio of the risk of occurrence of a disease among exposed people to that among the unexposed. As shown in Table 2.4, the risk ratio of stroke in women who smoke, compared with those who have never smoked, is 2.8 (49.6 /17.7).

The risk ratio is a better indicator of the strength of an association than the risk difference, because it is expressed relative to a baseline level of occurrence. Unlike the risk difference, it is related to the magnitude of the baseline incidence rate; populations with similar risk differences can have greatly differing risk ratios, depending on the magnitude of the baseline rates.

The risk ratio is used in assessing the likelihood that an association represents a causal relationship. For example, the risk ratio of lung cancer in long-term heavy smokers compared with non-smokers is approximately 20. This is very high and indicates that this relationship is not likely to be a chance finding. Of course, smaller risk ratios can also indicate a causal relationship, but care must be taken to eliminate other possible explanations (see Chapter 5).

Attributable risk

Attributable risk is the rate (proportion) of a disease or other outcome in exposed individuals that can be attributed to the exposure. This is a more useful term for public health purposes as it reflects the amount, usually expressed as a percentage, by which the risk of a disease is reduced by elimination or control of a particular exposure. Using attributable risk, it is possible to estimate the number of people spared the consequences of exposure, by subtracting the rate of the outcome (usually incidence or mortality) among the unexposed from the rate among the exposed individuals. For example, if there were 6 deaths per 100 among smokers, and 1 death per 100 in non-smokers, the attributable risk would be 5 per 100. This assumes that causes other than the one under investigation have had equal effects on the exposed and unexposed groups.

In summary, there are various measures for studying populations. Chapter 3 refers to many of these measures in the context of study design.

Study questions

2.1 What are the three epidemiological measures of disease frequency and how are they related?

2.2 Is prevalence rate a useful measure of the frequency of type 2 diabetes in different populations? What are the possible explanations for the variation in diabetes prevalence rates indicated in Table 2.3?

2.3 What is the population attributable risk or attributable fraction (proportion) for smokers in the example in Table 2.4?

2.4 What measures are used to compare the frequency of disease in populations and what information do they provide?

2.5 The relative risk of lung cancer associated with passive smoking is low, but the population attributable risk is considerable. What is the explanation for this?

2.6 What is the main reason for standardizing rates to a population with a standard age distribution (for example, the WHO world standard population)?

2.7 If you want to know where the most cancer deaths per capita occur within in a country, which is appropriate: crude death rates or age-standardized rates?

2.8 The crude death rate per 100 000 population for all cancers in Côte d'Ivoire is 70.5 and the age-standardized death rate is 160.2 per 100 000 population. What explains the large difference between these two rates?

2.9. The crude death rate for all cancers in Japan is 241.7 per 100 000 population and the crude death rate for all cancers in Côte d'Ivoire is 70.5 per 100 000 population. Is the death rate in Japan higher than that in Côte d'Ivoire?

References

1. *Constitution of the World Health Organization*. New York, World Health Organization, 1946.

2. Jong-wook L. Global health improvement and WHO: shaping the future. *Lancet* 2003;362:2083-8.

3. Torrence ME. *Understanding Epidemiology. Mosby's Biomedical Science Series*. Missouri, Mosby-Year Book Inc., 1997.

4. Special Writing Group of the Committee on Rheumatic Fever. Endocarditis, and Kawasaki Disease in the Young of the American Heart Association. Guidelines for the diagnosis of rheumatic fever. Jones criteria, 1992 update. *JAMA* 1992;268:2069-73.

5. *The management of acute respiratory infections in children. Practical guidelines for outpatient care*. Geneva, World Health Organization,1995.

6. *WHO recommended surveillance standards*. Geneva, World Health Organization. 1997.

7. Revised Classification System for HIV Infection and Expanded Surveillance Case Definition for AIDS Among Adolescents and Adults. *MMWR Recomm Rep* 1993;1992:41.

8. Prineas RJ, Crow RS, Blackburn H. *The Minnesota code manual of electrocardiographic findings: standards and procedures for measurement and classification*. Stoneham, MA, Butterworth Publications, 1982.

9. Luepker RV, Evans A, McKeigue P, Reddy KS. *Cardiovascular Survey Methods*, 3rd ed. Geneva, World Health Organization, 2004.

10. Alpert JS, Thygesen K, Antman E, Bassand JP. Myocardial infarction redefined— a consensus document of The Joint European Society of Cardiology/American College of Cardiology Committee for the redefinition of myocardial infarction. *J Am Coll Cardiol* 2000;36:959-69.

11. Last JM. *A dictionary of epidemiology*, 4th ed. Oxford, Oxford University Press, 2001.

12. King H, Rewers M. Global estimates for prevalence of diabetes mellitus and impaired glucose tolerance in adults. WHO Ad Hoc Diabetes Reporting Group. *Diabetes Care* 1993;16:157-77.

13. Colditz GA, Bonita R, Stampfer MJ, Willett WC, Rosner B, Speizer FE, et al. Cigarette smoking and risk of stroke in middle-aged women. *N Engl J Med* 1988;318:937-41.

14. International Statistical Classification of Diseases and Related Health Problems. *Tenth Revision. Vol. 1.* Geneva, World Health Organization, 1992.

15. Shibuya K. Counting the dead is essential for health. *Bull World Health Organ* 2006;84:170-1.

16. Shibuya K, Boerma T. Measuring progress towards reducing health inequalities. *Bull World Health Organ* 2005;83:162.

17. Mathers CD, Ma Fat D, Inoue M, Rao C, Lopez AD. Counting the dead and what they died from: an assessment of the global status of cause of death. *Bull World Health Organ* 2005;83:171-7.

18. *Population, Health and Survival at INDEPTH Sites. Vol 5.* Ottawa, The International Development Research Centre, 2002.

19. Sibai AM. Mortality certification and cause of death reporting in developing countries. *Bull World Health Organ* 2005;83:83.

20. Setel PW. Sample registration of vital events with verbal autopsy: a renewed commitment to measuring and monitoring vital statistics. *Bull World Health Organ* 2005;83:611-7.

21. Soleman N, Chandramohan D, Shibuya K. Verbal autopsy: current practices and challenges. *Bull World Health Organ* 2006;84:239-45.

22. Moser K, Shkolnikov V, Leon DA. World mortality 1950–2000: divergence replaces convergence from the late 1980s. *Bull World Health Organ* 2005;83:202-9.

23. *World Health Report 2005: Make every mother and child count.* Geneva, World Health Organization, 2005.

24. Feachem RGA, Kjellstrom T, Murray CJL, Over M, Phillips MA. *The health of adults in the developing world.* Oxford, Oxford University Press, 1992.

25. *World Health Statistics 2006.* Geneva, World Health Organization, 2006.

26. McKee M, Zatonski W. Public Health in Eastern Europe and the Former Soviet Union. In: Beaglehole R, ed. *Global Public Health: A New Era.* Oxford, Oxford University Press, 2003.

27. Barford A, Dorling D, Davey Smith G, Shaw M. Life expectancy: women now on top everywhere. *BMJ* 2006;332:808.

28. *World Health Report 2006: Working together for health.* Geneva, World Health Organization, 2006.

29. Waterhouse J. Muir, C., Correa, P., Powell, J. & Davis, W. *Cancer Incidence in Five Continents,* Vol. III. IARC Scient. Publ. 15. Lyon, IARC, 1976.

30. Ahmad OB, Boschi-Pinto C, Lopez AD, Murray CJL, Lozano R, Inoue M. *Age standardization of rates: a new WHO standard.* (GPE discussion paper series no. 31). Geneva, World Health Organization, 2001.

31. Lwanga SK, Tye CY, Ayeni O. *Teaching health statistics: lesson and seminar outlines,* 2nd ed. Geneva, World Health Organization, 1999.

32. *International classification of impairments, disabilities and handicaps. A manual of classification relating to the consequences of disease.* Geneva, World Health Organization, 1980.

33. Lee JW. Public health is a social issue. *Lancet* 2005;365:1005-6.

34. Irwin A, Valentine N, Brown C, Loewenson, R, Solar O, et al. The Commission on Social Determinants of Health: Tackling the social roots of health inequities. *PLoS Med* 2006;3:e106.

35. 35. Marmot M. Social determinants of health inequalities. *Lancet* 2005;365: 1099-104. Medline

36. Tunstall-Pedoe H, Vanuzzo D, Hobbs M, Mahonen M, Cepaitis Z, Kuulasmaa K, et al. Estimation of contribution of changes in coronary care to improving survival, event rates, and coronary heart disease mortality across the WHO MONICA Project populations. *Lancet* 2000;355:688-700.

37. Tolonen H, Dobson A, Kulathinal S, for the WHO MONICA Project. Assessing the quality of risk factor survey data: lessons from the WHO MONICA Project. *Eur J Cardiovasc Prev Rehab* 2005;13:104-14.

38. Armstrong T, Bonita R. Capacity building for an integrated noncommunicable disease risk factor surveillance system in developing countries. *Ethn Dis* 2003;13:S2-13.

39. Bonita R, Winkelmann R, Douglas KA, de Courten M. The WHO STEPwise approach to surveillance (STEPS) of noncommunicable disease risk factors. In: McQueen DV, Puska P, eds. *Global Risk Factor Surveillance.* New York, Kluwer Academic/Plenum Publishers, 2003:9–22.

40. Ezzati M, Lopez AD, Rodgers A, Murray CJL. *Comparative Quantification of Health Risks: Global and Regional Burden of Disease Attributable to Selected Major Risk Factors.* Geneva, World Health Organization, 2004.

41. World Bank. *World Development Report: Investing in Health.* Washington: World Bank, 1993.

42. *The World Health Report: Reducing Risks, Promoting Healthy Life.* Geneva, World Health Organization, 2002.

Chapter 3
Types of studies

Key messages

- Choosing the appropriate study design is a crucial step in an epidemiological investigation.
- Each study design has strengths and weaknesses.
- Epidemiologists must consider all sources of bias and confounding, and strive to reduce them.
- Ethical issues are important in epidemiology, as in other sciences.

Observations and experiments

Epidemiological studies can be classified as either observational or experimental. The most common types of study are listed with their alternative names and units of study in Table 3.1. The terms in the left-hand column are used throughout this book.

Observational studies

Observational studies allow nature to take its course: the investigator measures but does not intervene. They include studies that can be called descriptive or analytical:

- A **descriptive study** is limited to a description of the occurrence of a disease in a population and is often the first step in an epidemiological investigation.
- An **analytical study** goes further by analysing relationships between health status and other variables.

Apart from the simplest descriptive studies, almost all epidemiological studies are analytical in character. Pure descriptive studies are rare, but descriptive data in reports of health statistics are a useful source of ideas for epidemiological studies.

Limited descriptive information (such as that provided in a case series) in which the characteristics of several patients with a specific disease are described but are not compared with those of a reference population, often stimulates the initiation of a more detailed epidemiological study. For example, the description in 1981 of four young men with a previously rare form of pneumonia was the first in a wide range of epidemiological studies on the condition that became known as the acquired immunodeficiency syndrome (AIDS).[1]

Experimental studies

Experimental or intervention studies involve an active attempt to change a disease determinant – such as an exposure or a behaviour – or the progress of a disease through treatment, and are similar in design to experiments in other sciences. However, they

Table 3.1. Types of epidemiological study

Type of study	Alternative name	Unit of study
Observational studies		
Descriptive studies		
Analytical studies		
Ecological	Correlational	Populations
Cross-sectional	Prevalence	Individuals
Case-control	Case-reference	Individuals
Cohort	Follow-up	Individuals
Experimental studies	*Intervention studies*	
Randomized controlled trials	Clinical trials	Individuals
Cluster randomized controlled trials		Groups
Field trials		
Community trials	Community intervention studies	Healthy people Communities

are subject to extra constraints, since the health of the people in the study group may be at stake. Major experimental study designs include the following:

- randomized controlled trials using patients as subjects (clinical trials),
- field trials in which the participants are healthy people, and
- community trials in which the participants are the communities themselves.

In all epidemiological studies it is essential to have a clear definition of a case of the disease being investigated by delineating the symptoms, signs or other characteristics indicating that a person has the disease. A clear definition of an exposed person is also necessary. This definition must include all the characteristics that identify a person as being exposed to the factor in question. In the absence of clear definitions of disease and exposure, it is very difficult to interpret the data from an epidemiological study.

Observational epidemiology

Descriptive studies

A simple description of the health status of a community, based on routinely available data or on data obtained in special surveys as described in Chapter 2, is often the first step in an epidemiological investigation. In many countries this type of study is undertaken by a national centre for health statistics. Pure descriptive studies make no attempt to analyse the links between exposure and effect. They are usually based on mortality statistics and may examine patterns of death by age, sex or ethnicity during specified time periods or in various countries.

A classic example of descriptive data is shown in Figure 3.1, which charts the pattern of maternal mortality in Sweden since the middle of the eighteenth century, showing maternal death rates per 100 000 live births.[2] Such data can be of great value when identifying factors that have caused such a clear downward trend. It is

Figure 3.1. Maternal mortality rates in Sweden, 1750–1975[2]

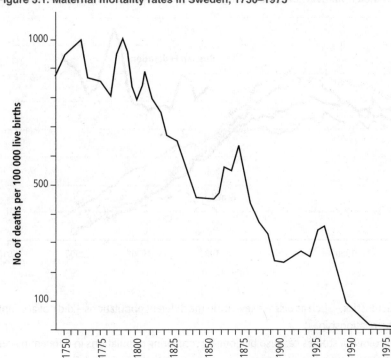

interesting to speculate on the possible changes in the living conditions of young women in the 1860s and 1870s which might have caused the temporary rise in maternal mortality at that time. In fact, this was a time of great poverty in Sweden and almost one million Swedes emigrated; most went to the United States of America.

Figure 3.2 is also based on routine death statistics and provides an example of the change in death rates of heart disease over time in six countries. It shows that death rates from heart disease have fallen by up to 70% in the last three decades in several countries, including Australia, Canada, the United Kingdom and the United States of America. Yet during the same time, the rates in other countries – such as Brazil and the Russian Federation – have remained the same or increased.[3] The next step in investigating this difference would require information about the comparability of the death certificates, changes in the incidence and case-fatality of the disease, and changes in the risk factors to which the relative populations have been exposed.

Ecological studies

Ecological (or correlational) studies are useful for generating hypotheses. In an ecological study, the units of analysis are groups of people rather than individuals. For example, a relationship was found between average sales of an anti-asthma drug and the occurrence of an unusually high number of asthma deaths in different provinces of New Zealand.[4] Such an observation would need to be tested by controlling for all the potential confounders to exclude the possibility that other

Figure 3.2. Age-standardized death rates from heart disease among men aged 30 years or more,[3] 1950–2002

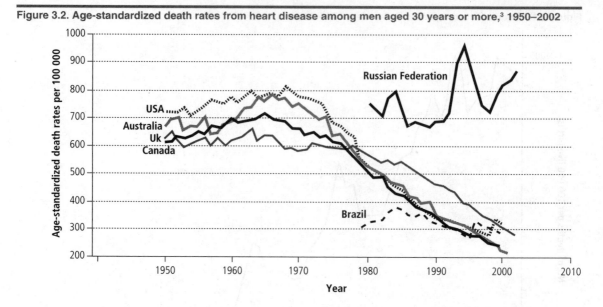

characteristics – such as disease severity in the different populations – did not account for the relationship.

Ecological studies can also be done by comparing populations in different places at the same time or, in a time series, by comparing the same population in one place at different times. Time series may reduce some of the socioeconomic confounding that is a potential problem in ecological studies. If the time period in a time series is very short, as it is in daily time series studies (Figure 3.3), confounding is virtually zero as the people in the study serve as their own controls.

Figure 3.3. Deaths during heat wave in Paris, 2003[5]

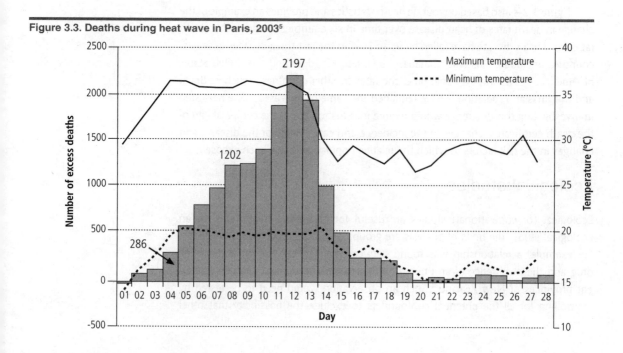

Although simple to conduct and thus attractive, ecological studies are often difficult to interpret since it is seldom possible to examine directly the various potential explanations for findings. Ecological studies usually rely on data collected for other purposes; data on different exposures and on socioeconomic factors may not be available. In addition, since the unit of analysis is a group, the link between exposure and effect at the individual level can not be made. One attraction of ecological studies is that data can be used from populations with widely differing characteristics or extracted from different data sources.

The increasing death rate during the heat wave in France in 2003 (Figure 3.3) correlated well with increasing temperature, although increasing daily air pollution also played a role. This increase of deaths occurred mainly among elderly people and the immediate cause of death was often recorded as heart or lung disease.

Ecological fallacy

An ecological fallacy or bias results if inappropriate conclusions are drawn on the basis of ecological data. The bias occurs because the association observed between variables at the group level does not necessarily represent the association that exists at the individual level (see Chapter 2). An example of a possible ecological fallacy is shown in Figure 3.4 in which an association is drawn between neonatal and maternal mortality and an absence of a skilled birth attendant.[6] Clearly many factors other than the presence of a skilled birth attendant impact on the outcome of a delivery. Such ecological inferences, however limited, can provide a fruitful start for more detailed epidemiological work.

Figure 3.4. Neonatal and maternal mortality are related to the absence of a skilled birth attendant.[6]

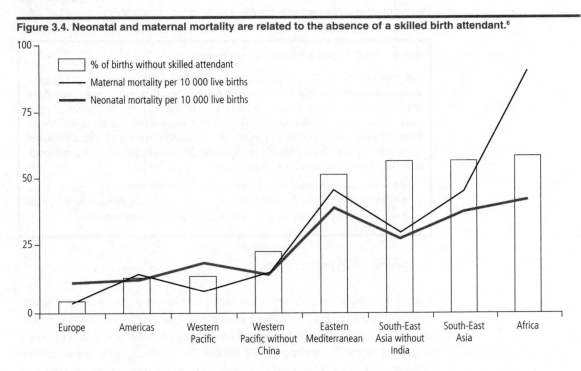

Cross-sectional studies

Cross-sectional studies measure the prevalence of disease and thus are often called prevalence studies. In a cross-sectional study the measurements of exposure and effect are made at the same time. It is not easy to assess the reasons for associations shown in cross-sectional studies. The key question to be asked is whether the exposure precedes or follows the effect. If the exposure data are known to represent exposure before any effect occurred, the data from a cross-sectional study can be treated like data generated from a cohort study.

Cross-sectional studies are relatively easy and inexpensive to conduct and are useful for investigating exposures that are fixed characteristics of individuals, such as ethnicity or blood group. In sudden outbreaks of disease, a cross-sectional study to measure several exposures can be the most convenient first step in investigating the cause.

Data from cross-sectional studies are helpful in assessing the health care needs of populations. Data from repeated cross-sectional surveys using independent random samples with standardized definitions and survey methods provide useful indications of trends.[7,8] Each survey should have a clear purpose. Valid surveys need well-designed questionnaires, an appropriate sample of sufficient size, and a good response rate.

Many countries conduct regular cross-sectional surveys on representative samples of their populations focusing on personal and demographic characteristics, illnesses and health-related habits. Frequency of disease and risk factors can then be examined in relation to age, sex and ethnicity. Cross-sectional studies of risk factors for chronic diseases have been done in a wide range of countries (Box 3.1)

Box 3.1. WHO Global InfoBase: an online tool

The WHO Global InfoBase (http://infobase.who.int) is a data warehouse that collects, stores and displays information on chronic diseases and their risk factors (overweight/obesity, blood pressure, cholesterol, alcohol, tobacco use, fruit/vegetable intake, physical inactivity, diabetes) for 186 countries. The InfoBase was initiated in 2002 to improve the access of health professionals and researchers to country-reported chronic disease risk factor data. It has the advantage of providing traceable sources and full survey methodology. The following options are available online:

- compare countries using WHO estimates for certain risk factors
- make country profiles showing the most recent most nationally-representative data
- use a survey search tool for all country data on particular risk factors

---

Case-control studies

Case-control studies provide a relatively simple way to investigate causes of diseases, especially rare diseases. They include people with a disease (or other outcome variable) of interest and a suitable control (comparison or reference) group of people unaffected by the disease or outcome variable. The study compares the occurrence of the possible cause in cases and in controls. The investigators collect data on disease occurrence at one point in time and exposures at a previous point in time.

Case-control studies are longitudinal, in contrast to cross-sectional studies (Figure 3.5). Case-control studies have been called retrospective studies since the investigator is looking backward from the disease to a possible cause. This can be confusing because the terms retrospective and prospective are also used to describe the timing of data collection in relation to the current date. In this sense a case-control study may be either retrospective, when all the data deal with the past, or prospective, in which data collection continues with the passage of time.

Figure 3.5. Design of a case-control study

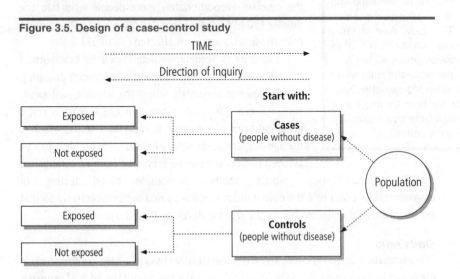

Direction of inquiry

TIME

Start with:

Exposed

Not exposed

Cases
(people without disease)

Population

Exposed

Not exposed

Controls
(people without disease)

Selection of cases and controls

A case-control study begins with the selection of cases; these cases should represent all the cases in a specified population group. Cases are selected on the basis of disease, not exposure. Controls are people without the disease. A critical and challenging aspect of population-based case control studies is finding a cost-effective way to identify and enroll control subjects.[9] The most difficult task is to select controls so as to sample the exposure prevalence in the population that generated the cases. Furthermore, the choice of controls and cases must not be influenced by exposure status, which should be determined in the same manner for both. It is not necessary for cases and controls to be all-inclusive; in fact they can be restricted to any specified subgroup, such as elderly people, males or females.

The controls should represent people who would have been designated study cases if they had developed the disease. Ideally, case-control studies use new (incident) cases to avoid the difficulty of separating factors related to causation and survival (or recovery), although studies have often been conducted using prevalence data (for example, case-control studies of congenital malformations). Case control studies can estimate relative risk of disease, but they can not determine the absolute incidence of disease.

Exposure

An important aspect of case-control studies is the determination of the start and duration of exposure for cases and controls. In the case-control design, the exposure status of the cases is usually determined after the development of the disease (retrospective data) and usually by direct questioning of the affected person or a relative or friend (Box 3.2). The informant's answers may be influenced by knowledge about the hypothesis under investigation or the disease experience itself.

An example of the use of a case-control study design is shown in Table 3.2. Researchers in Papua New Guinea compared the history of meat consumption in people who had enteritis necroticans, with people who did not have the disease. Proportionately more people who had the disease (50 of 61 cases) reported prior meat consumption than those who were not affected (16 of 57).[11]

Exposure is sometimes determined by biochemical measurements (e.g. lead in blood or cadmium in urine), which may not accurately reflect the relevant past exposure. For example, lead in blood at age 6 years is not a good indicator of exposure at age 1 to 2 years, which is the age of greatest sensitivity to lead. This problem can be avoided if exposure can be estimated from an established recording system (e.g. stored results of routine blood testing or employment records) or if the case-control study is carried out prospectively so that exposure data are collected before the disease develops (Box 3.3).

Box 3.2. Thalidomide

A classic example of a case-control study was the discovery of the relationship between thalidomide and limb defects in babies born in the Federal Republic of Germany in 1959 and 1960. The study, done in 1961, compared affected children with normal children. Of 46 mothers whose babies had malformations, 41 had been given thalidomide between the fourth and ninth weeks of pregnancy, whereas none of the 300 control mothers, whose children were normal, had taken the drug during pregnancy.[10] Accurate timing of the drug intake was crucial for determining relevant exposure.

Odds ratio

The association of an exposure and a disease (relative risk) in a case-control study is measured by calculating the odds ratio (OR), which is the ratio of the odds of exposure among the cases to the odds of exposure among the controls. For the data in Table 3.3, the odds ratio is given by:

$$OR = (50/11) \div (16/41) = \frac{50 \times 41}{11 \times 16} = 11.6$$

This indicates that the cases were 11.6 times more likely than the controls to have recently eaten meat.

The odds ratio is very similar to the risk ratio, particularly if a disease is rare. For the odds ratio to be a good approximation, the cases and controls must be representative of the general population with respect to exposure. However, because the incidence of disease is unknown, the absolute risk can not be calculated. An odds ratio should be accompanied by the confidence interval observed around the point estimate (see Chapter 4).

Table 3.2. Association between meat consumption and enteritis necroticans in Papua New Guinea[11]

		Exposure (recent meat ingestion)		
		Yes	No	Total
Disease (enteritis necroticans)	Yes	50	11	61
	No	16	41	57
	Total	66	52	118

Cohort studies

Cohort studies, also called follow-up or incidence studies, begin with a group of people who are free of disease, and who are classified into subgroups according to exposure to a potential cause of disease or outcome (Figure 3.6). Variables of interest are specified and measured and the whole cohort is followed up to see how the subsequent development of new cases of the disease (or other outcome) differs between the groups with and without exposure. Because the data on exposure and

Figure 3.6. Design of a cohort study

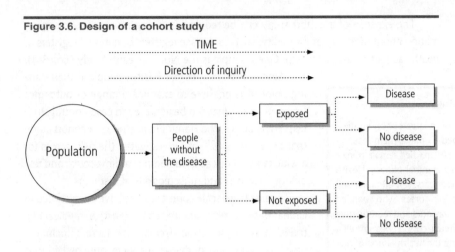

disease refer to different points in time, cohort studies are longitudinal, like case-control studies.

Cohort studies have been called prospective studies, but this terminology is confusing and should be avoided. As mentioned previously, the term "prospective" refers to the timing of data collection and not to the relationship between exposure and effect. Thus there can be both prospective and retrospective cohort studies.

Cohort studies provide the best information about the causation of disease and the most direct measurement of the risk of developing disease. Although conceptually simple, cohort studies are major undertakings and may require long periods of follow-up since disease may occur a long time after exposure. For example, the induction period for leukaemia or thyroid cancer caused by radiation (i.e. the time required for the specific cause to produce an outcome) is many years and it is necessary to follow up study par-ticipants for a long time. Many exposures investigated are long-term in nature and accurate information about them requires data collection over long periods. However, in the case of tobacco use, many people have relatively stable habits and information about past and current exposure can be collected at the time the cohort is defined.

In situations with sudden acute exposures, the cause-effect relationship for acute effects may be obvious, but cohort studies are also used to investigate late or chronic effects (Box 3.3).

> **Box 3.3. Late effects of poisoning: Bhopal**
>
> An example of measuring effects over a long time period is the catastrophic poisoning of residents around a pesticide factory in Bhopal, India, in 1984.[12] An intermediate chemical in the production process, methyl isocyanate, leaked from a tank and the fumes drifted into surrounding residential areas, exposing half a million people to the gas. 20 000 people died as a result of this exposure. In addition, 120 000 people still suffer health effects caused by the accident and subsequent pollution. The acute effects were easily studied with a cross-sectional design. More subtle chronic effects and those developing only after a long latency period are still being studied using cohort study designs.

As cohort studies start with exposed and unexposed people, the difficulty of measuring or finding existing data on individual exposures largely determines the feasibility of doing one of these studies. If the disease is rare in the exposed group as well as the unexposed group there may also be problems in obtaining a large enough study group.

The expense of a cohort study can be reduced by using routine sources information about mortality or morbidity, such as disease registers or national registers of deaths as part of the follow-up. One example is the Nurses Health Study (Box 3.4).

Since cohort studies take healthy people as their starting-point, it is possible to examine a range of outcomes (in contrast to what can be achieved in case-control studies). For example, the Framingham study – a cohort study that began in 1948 – has investigated the risk factors for a wide range of diseases, including cardiovascular and respiratory diseases and musculoskeletal disorders.[14]

Similar large-scale cohort studies have been started in China. Baseline demographic characteristics, medical histories, and major cardiovascular risk factors including blood pressure and body weight were obtained from a representative sample of 169 871 men and women 40 years of age and older in 1990. Researchers plan to follow this cohort on a regular basis.[15]

A special type of cohort study is the study of identical twins, where the confounding factor of genetic variation – between people exposed and not exposed to a particular factor – can be eliminated. Such studies have provided strong evidence for a variety of cause-effect relationships for chronic diseases. The Swedish twin registry is a good example of the type of data source that can be used to answer many epidemiological questions.[16]

Box 3.4. Nurses' Health Study

Although cost is a major factor in large cohort studies, methods have been developed to make them less expensive to run. In 1976, 121 700 married female nurses aged 30–55 years completed the initial Nurses' Health Survey questionnaire. Every two years, self-administered questionnaires were sent to these nurses, who supplied information on their health behaviours and reproductive and medical histories. The initial cohort was enrolled with the objective of evaluating the health effects of oral contraceptive use. Investigators tested their methods on small subgroups of the larger cohort, and obtained information on disease outcomes from routine data sources.[13] In addition to studying the relationship between oral contraceptive use and the risk of ovarian and breast cancer, they were also able to evaluate other diseases in this cohort – such as heart disease and stroke, and the relationship between smoking and the risk of stroke; as shown in Table 2.3. Although stroke is a relatively common cause of death, it is a rare occurrence in younger women, and so a large cohort is necessary.[10]

Historical cohort studies

Costs can occasionally be reduced by using a historical cohort (identified on the basis of records of previous exposure). This type of investigation is called a historical cohort study, because all the exposure and effect (disease) data have been collected before the actual study begins. For example, records of military personnel exposure to radioactive fall-out at nuclear bomb testing sites have been used to examine the possible causal role of fall-out in the development of cancer over the past 30 years.[17] This sort of design is relatively common for studies of cancer related to occupational exposures.

Nested case-control studies

The nested case-control design makes cohort studies less expensive. The cases and controls are both chosen from a defined cohort, for which some information on exposures and risk factors is already available (Figure 3.7). Additional information on new cases and controls, particularly selected for the study, is collected and analysed. This design is particularly useful when measurement of exposure is expensive. An example of a nested case control study is shown in Box 3.5.

Box 3.5. Nested case-control study of gastric cancer

To determine if infection with *Helicobacter pylori* was associated with gastric cancer, investigators used a cohort of 128 992 people that had been established in the mid-1960s. By 1991, 186 people in the original cohort had developed gastric cancer. The investigators then did a nested case-control study by selecting the 186 people with gastric cancer as cases and another 186 cancer-free individuals from the same cohort as controls. *H. pylori* infection status was determined retrospectively from serum samples that had been stored since the 1960s. 84% of people with gastric cancer – and only 61% of the controls – had been infected previously with *H. pylori,* suggesting a positive association between *H. pylori* infection and gastric cancer risk.[18]

Figure 3.7. Design of a nested case-control study

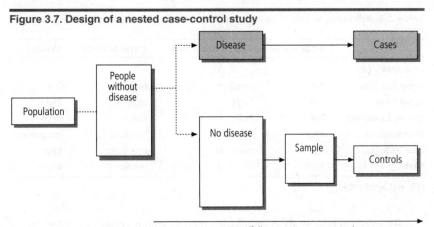

Time (follow-up over many years)

Summary of epidemiological studies

Table 3.3 summarizes the applications of different observational studies and Table 3.4 outlines the advantages and disadvantages of the major types of observational study.

Table 3.3. Applications of different observational study designs [a]

Objective	Ecological	Cross-sectional	Case-control	Cohort
Investigation of rare disease	++++	−	+++++	−
Investigation of rare cause	++	−	−	+++++
Testing multiple effects of cause	+	++	−	+++++
Study of multiple exposures and determinants	++	++	++++	+++
Measurements of time relationship	++	−	+ [b]	+++++
Direct measurement of incidence	−	−	+ [c]	+++++
Investigation of long latent periods	−	−	+++	−

[a] +...+++++ indicates the general degree of suitability; there are exceptions
− not suitable.
[b] If prospective.
[c] If population-based.

Experimental epidemiology

Intervention or experimentation involves attempting to change a variable in one or more groups of people. This could mean the elimination of a dietary factor thought to cause allergy, or testing a new treatment on a selected group of patients. The effects of an intervention are measured by comparing the outcome in the experimental group with that in a control group. Since the interventions are strictly determined by the study protocol, ethical considerations are of paramount importance in the design of these studies. For example, no patient should be denied appropriate treatment as a result of participation in an experiment, and the treatment being tested must be acceptable in the light of current knowledge. Informed consent from study participants is required in almost all circumstances.

Table 3.4. Advantages and disadvantages of different observational study designs

	Ecological	Cross-sectional	Case-control	Cohort
Probability of:				
selection bias	NA	medium	high	low
recall bias	NA	high	high	low
loss to follow-up	NA	NA	low	high
confounding	High	medium	medium	medium
time required	Low	medium	medium	high
cost	Low	medium	medium	high

NA: not applicable.

An interventional study is usually designed as a randomized controlled trial, a field trial, or a community trial.

Randomized controlled trials

A randomized controlled trial is an epidemiological experiment designed to study the effects of a particular intervention. Subjects in the study population are randomly allocated to intervention and control groups, and the results are assessed by comparing outcomes.

The design of a randomized controlled trial is shown in Figure 3.8. To ensure that the groups being compared are equivalent, patients are allocated to them randomly, i.e. by chance. If the initial selection and randomization is done properly, the control and treatment groups will be comparable at the start of the investigation; any differences between groups are chance occurrences unaffected by the conscious or unconscious biases of the investigators.

Figure 3.8. Design of a randomized controlled trial

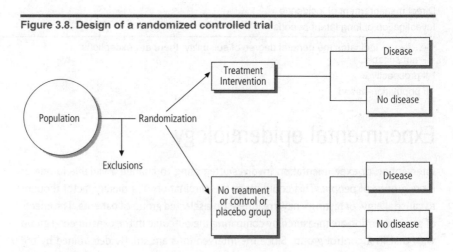

Field trials

Field trials, in contrast to clinical trials, involve people who are healthy but presumed to be at risk; data collection takes place "in the field," usually among non-institutionalized people in the general population. Since the subjects are disease-free and the purpose is to prevent diseases that may occur with relatively low frequency, field trials are often logistically complicated and expensive endeavours. One of the largest field trials was that testing the Salk vaccine for the prevention of poliomyelitis, which involved over one million children.

Field trials can be used to evaluate interventions aimed at reducing exposure without necessarily measuring the occurrence of health effects. For instance, different protective methods for pesticide exposure have been tested in this way and measurement of blood lead levels in children has shown the protection provided by elimination of lead paint in the home environment. Such intervention studies can be done on a smaller scale, and at lower cost, as they do not involve lengthy follow-up or measurement of disease outcomes.

Community trials

In this form of experiment, the treatment groups are communities rather than individuals. This is particularly appropriate for diseases that are influenced by social conditions, and for which prevention efforts target group behaviour. Cardiovascular disease is a good example of a condition appropriate for community trials although unanticipated methodological issues can arise in large community intervention trials (Box 3.6).

Limitations of community trials

A limitation of such studies is that only a small number of communities can be included and random allocation of communities is usually not practicable; other methods are required to ensure that any differences found at the end of the study can be attributed to the intervention rather than to inherent differences between communities.[19] Furthermore, it is difficult to isolate the communities where intervention is taking place from general social changes that may be occurring. Design limitations, especially in the face of unexpectedly large, favourable risk factor changes

> **Box 3.6. Stanford Five-City Community Intervention Trial**
>
> The Stanford Five-City Project started in 1978 as one of several community intervention studies designed to lower population risk of cardiovascular disease. Researchers believed that the community approach was the best way to address the large compounded risk of mild elevations of multiple risk factors and the interrelation of several health behaviours. Although some components of the intervention proved effective when evaluated individually (for example, efficiency of the mass media and other community-wide programs), large, favourable changes in risk factor also occurred in the control sites. Part of the problem was related to design limitations. Internal validity was compromised by the fact that only a few intervention units could be studied in sufficient detail. Researchers also noted the need to improve educational interventions and expand the environmental and health policy components of health promotion.[19]

in control sites, are difficult to overcome. As a result, definitive conclusions about the overall effectiveness of the community-wide efforts are not always possible.[20]

Figure 3.9 shows a community trial of a tuberculosis outreach programme in rural Ethiopia.[21] 32 communities – with a combined population of 350 000 people – were randomly allocated to intervention and control groups. The study showed that community outreach improved the speed of case-finding for smear-positive tuberculosis.

Potential errors in epidemiological studies

Epidemiological investigations aim to provide accurate measures of disease occurrence (or other outcomes). However, there are many possibilities for errors in measurement. Epidemiologists devote much attention to minimizing errors and assessing the impact of errors that can not be eliminated. Sources of error can be random or systematic.

Figure 3.9. Trial profile of communities randomized to intervention and control[23]

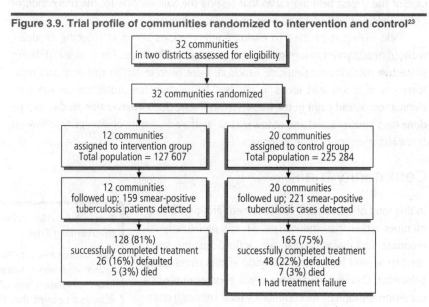

Random error

Random error is when a value of the sample measurement diverges – due to chance alone – from that of the true population value. Random error causes inaccurate measures of association. There are three major sources of random error:

- individual biological variation;
- sampling error; and
- measurement error.

Random error can never be completely eliminated since we can study only a sample of the population. Sampling error is usually caused by the fact that a small sample is not representative of all the population's variables. The best way to reduce sampling error is to increase the size of the study. Individual variation always occurs and no measurement is perfectly accurate. Measurement error can be reduced by stringent protocols, and by making individual measurements as precise as possible. Investigators need to understand the measurement methods being used in the study, and the errors that these methods can cause. Ideally, laboratories should be able to document the accuracy and precision of their measurements by systematic quality control procedures.

Sample size

The sample size must be large enough for the study to have sufficient statistical power to detect the differences deemed important. Sample size calculations can be done with standard formulae as provided in Chapter 4. The following information is needed before the calculation can be done:

- required level of statistical significance of the ability to detect a difference
- acceptable error, or chance of missing a real effect
- magnitude of the effect under investigation
- amount of disease in the population
- relative sizes of the groups being compared.

In reality, sample size is often determined by logistic and financial considerations, and a compromise always has to be made between sample size and costs. A practical guide to determining sample size in health studies has been published by WHO.[22]

The precision of a study can also be improved by ensuring that the groups are of appropriate relative size. This is often an issue of concern in case-control studies when a decision is required on the number of controls to be chosen for each case. It is not possible to be definitive about the ideal ratio of controls to cases, since this depends on the relative costs of accumulating cases and controls. If cases are scarce and controls plentiful, it is appropriate to increase the ratio of controls to cases. For example, in the case-control study of the effects of thalidomide (Box 3.2), 46 affected children were compared with 300 normal children. In general, however, there may be little point in having more than four controls for each case. It is important to ensure that there is sufficient similarity between cases and controls when the data are to be analysed by, for example, age group or social class; if most cases and only a few controls were in the older age groups, the study would not be able to account for the confounding factor of age.

Systematic error

Systematic error (or bias) occurs in epidemiology when results differ in a systematic manner from the true values. A study with a small systematic error is said to have a high accuracy. Accuracy is not affected by sample size.

The possible sources of systematic error in epidemiology are many and varied; over 30 specific types of bias have been identified. The principal biases are:

- selection bias
- measurement (or classification) bias.

Selection bias

Selection bias occurs when there is a systematic difference between the characteristics of the people selected for a study and the characteristics of those who are not. An obvious source of selection bias occurs when participants select themselves for a study, either because they are unwell or because they are particularly worried about an exposure. It is well known, for example, that people who respond to an invitation to participate in a study on the effects of smoking differ in their smoking habits from non-responders; the latter are usually heavier smokers. In studies of children's health, where parental cooperation is required, selection bias may also occur. In a cohort study of newborn children,[23] successful 12-month follow-up varied according to income level of the parents. If individuals entering or remaining in a study have different characteristics from those who are not selected initially, or who drop out before completion, the result is a biased estimate of the association between exposure and outcome.

An important selection bias is introduced when the disease or factor under investigation itself makes people unavailable for study. For example, in a factory where workers are exposed to formaldehyde, those who suffer most from eye irritation are most likely to leave their jobs. The remaining workers are less affected and a prevalence study of the association between formaldehyde exposure and eye irritation that is done only in the workplace may be very misleading.

In such occupational epidemiology studies this important selection bias is called the healthy worker effect (Chapter 9). Workers have to be healthy enough to perform their duties; the severely ill and disabled are usually excluded from employment. Similarly, if a study is based on examinations done in a health centre and there is no follow-up of participants who do not turn up, biased results may be produced: unwell patients may be in bed either at home or in hospital. All epidemiological study designs need to account for selection bias.

Measurement bias

Measurement bias occurs when the individual measurements or classifications of disease or exposure are inaccurate – that is, they do not measure correctly what they are supposed to measure. There are many sources of measurement bias and their effects are of varying importance. For instance, biochemical or physiological measurements are never completely accurate and different laboratories often produce different results on the same specimen. If specimens from the exposed and control groups are analysed randomly by different laboratories, there is less chance for systematic measurement bias than in the situation where all specimens from the exposed group are analysed in one laboratory and all those from the control group are analysed in another.

A form of measurement bias of particular importance in retrospective case-control studies is known as recall bias. This occurs when there is a differential recall of information by cases and controls; for instance, cases may be more likely to recall past exposure, especially if it is widely known to be associated with the disease under study – for example, lack of exercise and heart disease. Recall bias can either exaggerate the degree of effect associated with the exposure – as with people affected by heart disease being more likely to admit to a past lack of exercise – or underestimate it – if cases are more likely than controls to deny past exposure.

If measurement bias occurs equally in the groups being compared, it almost always results in an underestimate of the true strength of the relationship. Such non-differential bias may account for apparent discrepancies in the results of different epidemiological studies.

If the investigator, laboratory technician or the participant knows the exposure status, this knowledge can influence measurements and cause *observer bias*. To avoid this bias, measurements can be made in a *blind* or *double-blind* fashion. A blind study means that the investigators do not know how participants are classified.

A double-blind study means that neither the investigators, nor the participants, know how the latter are classified.

Confounding

Confounding is another major issue in epidemiological studies. In a study of the association between exposure to a cause (or risk factor) and the occurrence of disease, confounding can occur when another exposure exists in the study population and is associated both with the disease and the exposure being studied. A problem arises if this extraneous factor – itself a determinant or risk factor for the health outcome – is unequally distributed between the exposure subgroups. Confounding occurs when the effects of two exposures (risk factors) have not been separated and the analysis concludes that the effect is due to one variable rather than the other. To be a confounding factor, two conditions must be met (Figure 3.10).

Figure 3.10. Confounding: relationship between coffee drinking (exposure), heart disease (outcome), and a third variable (tobacco use)

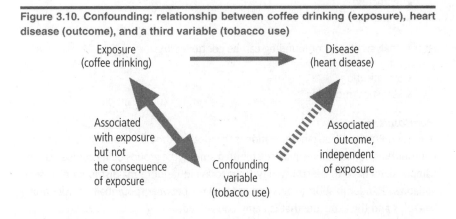

Confounding arises because non-random distribution of risk factors in the source population also occurs in the study population thus providing misleading estimates of effect (see Box 3.7). In this sense, it might appear to be a bias, but in fact it does not result from systematic error in research design.[25]

Age and social class are often confounders in epidemiological studies. An association between high blood pressure and coronary heart disease may in truth represent concomitant changes in the two variables that occur with increasing age; the potential confounding effect of age has to be considered, and when this is done it is seen that high blood pressure indeed increases the risk of coronary heart disease.

In the example in Figure 3.10, confounding may be the explanation for the relationship demonstrated between coffee drinking and the risk of coronary heart disease, since it is known that coffee consumption is associated with tobacco use: people who drink coffee are more likely to smoke than people who do not drink coffee.

Box 3.7. Confounding: difficult to control

The word "confounding" comes from the Latin *confundere*, meaning *to mix together*. Confounding can have a very important influence, and may even change the apparent direction of an association. A variable that appears to be protective may, after control of confounding, be found to be harmful. The most common concern about confounding is that it may create the appearance of a cause-effect relationship that does not actually exist. For a variable to be a confounder, it must, in its own right, be a determinant of the occurrence of disease (i.e. a risk factor) and associated with the exposure under investigation. Thus, in a study of radon exposure and lung cancer, smoking is not a confounder if the smoking habits are identical in the radon-exposed and control groups.

It is also well known that cigarette smoking is a cause of coronary heart disease. It is thus possible that the relationship between coffee drinking and coronary heart disease merely reflects the known causal association of tobacco use and heart disease. In this situation, smoking confounds the apparent relationship between coffee consumption and coronary heart disease because smoking is correlated with coffee drinking and is a risk factor even for those who do not drink coffee.

The control of confounding

Several methods are available to control confounding, either through study design or during the analysis of results.

The methods commonly used to control confounding in the design of an epidemiological study are:

- randomization
- restriction
- matching.

At the analysis stage, confounding can be controlled by:

- stratification
- statistical modeling.

Randomization

In experimental studies, randomization is the ideal method for ensuring that potential confounding variables are equally distributed among the groups being compared. The sample sizes have to be sufficiently large to avoid random maldistribution of such variables. Randomization avoids the association between potentially confounding variables and the exposure that is being considered.

Restriction

One way to control confounding is to limit the study to people who have particular characteristics. For example, in a study on the effects of coffee on coronary heart disease, participation in the study could be restricted to nonsmokers, thus removing any potential effect of confounding by cigarette smoking.

Matching

Matching is used to control confounding by selecting study participants so as to ensure that potential confounding variables are evenly distributed in the two groups being compared. For example, in a case-control study of exercise and coronary heart disease, each patient with heart disease can be matched with a control of the same age group and sex to ensure that confounding by age and sex does not occur. Matching has been used extensively in case-control studies but it can lead to problems in the selection of controls if the matching criteria are too strict or too numerous; this is called overmatching.

Matching can be expensive and time-consuming, but is particularly useful if the danger exists of there being no overlap between cases and controls, such as in a situation where the cases are likely to be older than the controls.

Stratification

In large studies it is usually preferable to control for confounding in the analytical phase rather than in the design phase. Confounding can then be controlled by *stratification*, which involves the measurement of the strength of associations in well defined and homogeneous categories (strata) of the confounding variable. If age is a confounder, the association may be measured in, say, 10-year age groups; if sex or ethnicity is a confounder, the association is measured separately in men and women or in the different ethnic groups. Methods are available for summarizing the overall association by producing a weighted average of the estimates calculated in each separate stratum.

Although stratification is conceptually simple and relatively easy to carry out, it is often limited by the size of the study and it can not help to control many factors simultaneously, as is often necessary. In this situation, multivariate statistical *modeling* is required to estimate the strength of the associations while controlling for several confounding variables simultaneously; a range of statistical techniques is available for these analyses (Chapter 4).

Validity

Validity is an expression of the degree to which a test is capable of measuring what it is intended to measure. A study is valid if its results correspond to the truth; there should be no systematic error and the random error should be as small as possible. Figure 3.11 indicates the relationship between the true value and measured values for low and high validity and reliability. With low reliability but high validity the measured values are spread out, but the mean of the measured values is close to the true value. On the other hand, a high reliability (or repeatability) of the measurements does not ensure validity since they may all be far from the true value. There are two types of validity: internal and external.

Figure 3.11. Validity and reliability

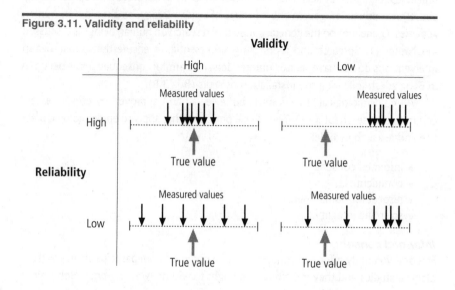

Internal validity

Internal validity is the degree to which the results of an observation are correct for the particular group of people being studied. For example, measurements of blood haemoglobin must distinguish accurately participants with anaemia as defined in the study. Analysis of the blood in a different laboratory may produce different results because of systematic error, but the evaluation of associations with anaemia, as measured by one laboratory, may still be internally valid.

For a study to be of any use it must be internally valid, although even a study that is perfectly valid internally may be of no consequence because the results can not be compared with other studies. Internal validity can be threatened by all sources of systematic error but can be improved by good design and attention to detail.

External validity

External validity or generalizability is the extent to which the results of a study apply to people not in it (or, for example, to laboratories not involved in it). Internal validity is necessary for, but does not guarantee, external validity, and is easier to achieve. External validity requires external quality control of the measurements and judgements about the degree to which the results of a study can be extrapolated. This does not require that the study sample be representative of a reference population. For example, evidence that the effect of lowering blood cholesterol in men is also relevant to women requires a judgment about the external validity of studies in men. External validity is assisted by study designs that examine clearly-stated hypotheses in well defined populations. The external validity of a study is supported if similar results are found in studies in other populations.[24]

Ethical issues

Ethical issues are those involving actions and policies that are right or wrong, fair or unfair, just or unjust. Ethical dilemmas arise frequently in the practice of epidemiology and ethical principles govern the conduct of epidemiology, as they do all human activities. Guidelines on the general conduct of research on human beings is discussed in Chapter 11. Research and monitoring are essential to ensure that public health interventions do not have serious unintended and harmful consequences as occurred in Bangladesh following the installation of wells (Box 3.8).

All epidemiological studies must be reviewed and approved by ethical review committees (see Chapter 11). The ethical principles that apply to epidemiologic practice and research include:

- informed consent
- confidentiality
- respect for human rights
- scientific integrity.

Informed consent

Free and voluntary informed consent must be obtained from participants in epidemiological studies and they must retain the right to withdraw at any time. However, it may prove impracticable for informed consent to be given for access to routine medical records. In such cases, as is the norm in any other research study, epidemiologists

---

Box 3.8. Unintended consequences: arsenic in tube wells in Bangladesh

The installation of tube wells to improve rural standards of water and hygiene in Bangladesh over the past few decades, has been an important element in the control of cholera and other waterborne enteric diseases. Although 95% of the population now relies on ground-water from these wells, no testing for microbial counts, heavy metals or toxic chemicals was carried out in the initial stages. It was only in 1985 when a local physician in West Bengal, India, began noticing patients with clinical signs of arsenic intoxication (skin pigmentation and increased rates of a variety of cancers), that the tube wells were checked. Currently about 30 million people, one quarter of Bangladesh's population, are drinking water with significantly high levels of arsenic. All of the possible interventions to lower arsenic intake from water (treating water at the pump, in-home treatment of water, community level water treatment, sealing wells with high arsenic content, and sinking deeper wells below the water table with high arsenic content) are either costly or require continuing maintenance and monitoring.[25] To date, there has been no national program to reduce tube well arsenic levels.[26]

---

must respect personal privacy and confidentiality at all times. They have an obligation to tell communities what they are doing and why, and to transmit the results of studies, and their significance, to the communities involved. All proposals for epidemiological studies should be submitted to properly constituted institutional ethics committees before the research work begins.

Confidentiality

Epidemiologists also have an obligation to preserve confidentiality of information they obtain through their studies. This also extends to the right of a person to withhold information from others. As information in medical records, case registers, and other data files and databases are generally confidential, epidemiologists are required to obtain permission before being given access to these data.

Respect for individual rights

Tension can often arise in epidemiological studies between the interests of the group and the interests of the individual. An example is provided by efforts to limit the public health impact of HIV/AIDS. Cuba successfully contained the spread of HIV/AIDS by testing individuals at risk and segregating infected people from the general population.[27] Others argue that individual human rights are key to preventing infection because spread of disease was facilitated by their denial; for example, women in many affected countries cannot refuse demands for unprotected sex. In addition, much of the behaviour that places individuals at risk of HIV/AIDS happens in private, beyond the reach of the state. Public health efforts to modify the behaviour of vulnerable people are unlikely to be successful without assurances that their interests will be protected.

Scientific integrity

All scientists have the potential to behave in an unethical manner, perhaps in part because of the pressure to succeed. Epidemiologists are not immune to unethical behaviour. Examples include research results apparently influenced by conflict of interests and the publication of fabricated data.[28, 29] Minimization of unethical behaviour requires vigilance on the part of ethical review committees and close

attention to peer review of publications.[30] The training and mentoring of epidemiologists must include serious and repeated discussion of these issues.

Study questions

3.1   What are the applications and disadvantages of the major epidemiological
       study designs?
3.2   Outline the design of a case-control study and a cohort study to examine the
       association of a high-fat diet with bowel cancer.
3.3   What is random error and how can it be reduced?
3.4   What are the main types of systematic error in epidemiological studies and
       how can their effects be reduced?
3.5   Describe in which studies the relative risk (RR) and the odds ratio (OR) are
       used. Outline the reasons why they would be used in a particular study and
       not in another.
3.6   In the case of a rare disease, the OR and RR can have very similar values.
       Explain the reasons behind this similarity.
3.7   A cross-sectional study of Downs syndrome has found an association with
       birth order. What could be a cause of confounding and how would you
       avoid it?

References

1. Gottlieb MS, Schroff R, Schanker HM, Weisman JD, Fan PT, Wolf RA, et al.
    Pneumocystis carinii pneumonia and mucosal candidiasis in previously healthy
    homosexual men: evidence of a new acquired cellular immunodeficiency.
    N Engl J Med 1981;305:1425-31.
2. Högberg U, Wall S. Secular trends in maternal mortality in Sweden from 1750
    to 1980. *Bull World Health Organ* 1986;64:79-84.
3. *Prevention of chronic diseases: a vital investment.* Geneva, World Health
    Organization, 2005.
4. Pearce N, Hensley MJ. Beta agonists and asthma deaths. *Epidemiol Rev*
    1998;20:173-86.
5. *Impact de la vague de chaleur.* Paris, Institute de Veille Sanitaire, 2003.
    http://www.invs.sante.fr/publications/2003/chaleur_aout_2003/rap_chaleur_
    290803.pdf
6. *World Health Report 2005: Make every mother and child count.* Geneva, World
    Health Organization, 2005.
7. Tolonen H, Dobson A, Kulathinal S, Sangita A, for the WHO MONICA
    Project. Assessing the quality of risk factor survey data: lessons from
    the WHO MONICA Project. *Eur J Cardiovasc Prev Rehabil* 2006;13:104-14.
8. Bonita R, Douglas K, Winkelmann R, De Courten M. The WHO STEPwise
    approach to surveillance (STEPS) of noncommunicable disease risk factors. In
    McQueen DV, Puska P eds. *Global Risk Factor Surveillance.* London, Kluwer
    Academic/Plenum Publishers, 2003:9-22.
9. Bernstein L. Control recruitment in population-based case-control studies.
    Epidemiology 2006;17:255-7.

10. Mellin GW, Katzenstein M. The saga of thalidomide. Neuropathy to embryopathy, with case reports of congenital anomalies. *N Engl J Med* 1962;267:1238-44.

11. Millar JS, Smellie S, Coldman AJ. Meat consumption as a risk factor in enteritis necroticans. *Int J Epidemiol* 1985;14:318-21.

12. Lapierre D, Moro J. *Five past midnight in Bhopal.* Warner Books, 2002.

13. Colditz GA, Martin P, Stampfer MJ, Willett WC, Sampson L, Rosner B, et al. Validation of questionnaire information on risk factors and disease outcomes in a prospective cohort study of women. *Am J Epidemiol* 1986;123:894-900.

14. Lloyd-Jones DM, Leip EP, Larson MG, D'Agostino RB, Beiser A, Wilson PW. Prediction of lifetime risk for cardiovascular disease by risk factor burden at 50 years of age. *Circulation* 2006;113:791-8.

15. Chen Z, Lee L, Chen J, Collins R, Wu F, Guo Y, et al. Cohort Profile: The Kadoorie Study of Chronic Disease in China (KSCDC). *Int J Epidemiol* 2005;34:1243-9.

16. Lichtenstein P, De Faire U, Floderus B, Svartengren M, Svedberg P, Pedersen NL. The Swedish twin registry: a unique resource for clinical, epidemiological and genetic studies. *J Intern Med* 2002;252:184-205.

17. Johnson JC, Thaul S, Page WF, Crawford H. *Mortality Of Veteran Participants In The Crossroads Nuclear Test.* Washington, National Academy Press, 1996.

18. Parsonnet J, Friedman GD, Vandersteen DP, Chang Y, Vogelman JH, Orentreich N, et al. Helicobacter pylori infection and the risk of gastric cancer. *N Engl J Med* 1991;325:1127-31.

19. Fortmann SP, Flora JA, Winkleby MA, Schooler C, Taylor CB, Farquhar JW. Community intervention trials: reflections on the Stanford Five-City Project Experience. *Am J Epidemiol* 1995;142:576-86.

20. Susser M. The tribulations of trials—interventions in communities. *Am J Public Health* 1995;85:156.

21. Shargie EB, Morkve O, Lindtjorn B. Tuberculosis case-finding through a village outreach programme in a rural setting in southern Ethiopia: community randomized trial. *Bull World Health Organ* 2006;84:112-9.

22. Lwanga SK, Lemeshow S. *Sample size determination in health studies.* Geneva, World Health Organization, 1991.

23. Victora CG, Barros FC, Vaughan JP, Teixeira AM. Birthweight and infant mortality: a longitudinal study of 5,914 Brazilian children. *Int J Epidemiol* 1987;16:239-45.

24. Grimes DA, Schulz KF. Bias and causal associations in observational research. *Lancet* 2002;359:248-52.

25. Smith AH, Lingas EO, Rahman, M. Contamination of drinking water by arsenic in Bangladesh: a public health emergency. *Bull World Health Organ* 2000;78:1093-3.

26. Pepper D. Bangladeshis poisoned by arsenic sue British organization. *Lancet* 2006;367:199-200.

27. Zipperer M. HIV/AIDS prevention and control: the Cuban response. *Lancet Infect Dis* 2005;5:400.

28. Wikler D, Cash R. Ethical issues in global public health. In Beaglehole R, ed. *Global Public Health: A New Era.* Oxford, Oxford University Press, 2003.

29. Horton R. Expression of concern: non-steroidal anti-inflammatory drugs and the risk of oral cancer. *Lancet* 2006;3167:1961.

30. Gollogly L, Momen H. Ethical dilemmas in scientific publication: pitfalls and solutions for editors. *Rev Saude Publica* 2006;40:24-30.

Chapter 4
Basic biostatistics: concepts and tools

O. Dale Williams

Key messages

- Basic epidemiology requires a knowledge of biostatistics.
- Good quality tables and graphs provide effective means of communicating data.
- Confidence intervals are valuable estimation tools and can be used to test hypotheses.
- Although calculations can be complex, the concepts underlying statistical tests are often quite simple.

Biostatistical concepts and tools are needed for summarizing and analysing data.[1-5] Doing and interpreting epidemiological research requires the use of samples to make inferences about populations. This chapter will describe basic concepts and methods, and how to summarize data.

In the event that students wish more details on these basic concepts, there are numerous online courses and texts freely available; see Chapter 11 for some suggestions.

Before describing the basic concepts and tools, it is useful to become familiar with the various methods for interpreting and communicating data. This section is intended to provide the most common ways of summarizing data; examples in other chapters are used to illustrate the general principles.

Summarizing data

Data exist as either numerical or categorical variables.

- Numerical variables include counts, such as the number of children of a specific age, and measurements, such as height and weight.
- Categorical variables are the result of classifying. For instance, individuals can be classified into categories according to their blood group; A, B, O, or AB. Ordinal data – which express ranks – are a type of categorical data.

Tables and graphs can be used for summarizing data. Summary numbers include medians, means, ranges, standard deviations, standard errors and variances. These are explained below, along with suggestions and cautions as to their appropriate use.

Tables and graphs

Tables and graphs are important means of summarizing and displaying data, but they are seldom prepared with sufficient care. Their purpose is to display data in a way that can be quickly and easily understood. *Each table or graph should contain enough information so that it can be interpreted without reference to the text.*

Titles play a critical role in making a table or graph useful to the reader. Titles should specifically describe the numbers included in the cells of a table or represented by the points plotted on a graph. For tables, the title should clearly state what the numbers in the cell represent, how the cells are classified, and where and when the data were collected. A common problem is for the title to state the purpose of the table or graph rather than to describe what it contains.

Epidemiologists often have to decide how to present data and whether to choose a table or a graph. While these two share some common features, one is likely to be more suitable than the other in specific cases (Box 4.1).

There are several types of graphs to consider. Here are some of the more popular, along with some guidance on their use.

Box 4.1. The advantages of graphs versus tables

Graphs have the advantages of:

- simplicity and clarity
- memorable visual images
- being able to show complex relationships.

They also emphasize numbers and tend to be popular, as evidenced by their use in general publications where tables are rarely used.

Tables have the advantages of:

- displaying more complex data with precision and flexibility
- requiring less technical skill or facilities to prepare
- using less space for a given amount of information.

Box 4.2. World health chart

The world health chart (http://www.gapminder.org/) shows global health development by a series of interactive charts linked to existing data. These charts are designed to promote better use of such data, inform advocacy efforts and stimulate hypothesis generation. The charts show time trends in a dynamic fashion, similar to a computer game. The world health chart can help to answer questions such as:

- How do wealth and health relate historically?
- Has the world become healthier over the past 50-100 years?
- How have the differences in health between countries changed?

Pie charts and component band charts

Pie charts (Figure 6.2) and component band charts (Figure 2.3) display how a whole entity is divided into its parts. A pie chart represents this information with a circle and a component band chart represents it with a bar – both are divided into sections representing the different components. For pie charts, a useful rule is to place the pieces of the pie in order according to their size, starting at the equivalent of twelve o'clock and then progressing clockwise. In general, it is better to use component band charts for comparing how two or more whole entities are divided into their component parts than it is to place pie charts side by side.

Spot maps and rate maps

Spot maps and rate maps display geographical locations of cases or rates. John Snow used this spot map to display where the cases of cholera occurred relative to the famous pump (Figure 4.1). Rate maps are slightly different in that geographical areas are shaded according the differences in values; prevalence, incidence or mortality are often shown on rate maps. Areas with the highest rates are typically shaded with the darkest shades or the brightest colors (Figure 4.2).

Figure 4.1. Deaths from cholera in central London, September 1854[6,7]

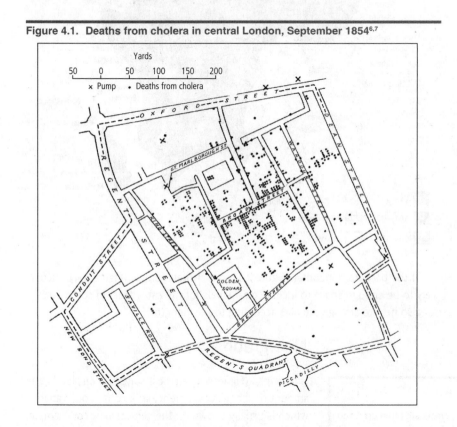

Maps, charts, and atlases are used to display data in both a static form – such as in the Mental Health Atlas, the Tobacco Atlas, and the Cancer Atlas – and in an interactive form (Box 4.3), but these will not be discussed further in this chapter. A free online course for use of interactive maps based on data from the Human Development Report can be found at http://hdr.undp.org/statistics/data/animation.cfm.

Bar charts

Bar charts are best suited for displaying numbers or percentages that compare two or more categories of data, such as the proportions of male to female smokers. The lengths of the bars convey the essence of this comparison so that any alterations or distortions of these lengths – such as scale breaks – are usually inappropriate (Box 4.3).

Figure 4.2. Under-five mortality per 1000 live births in African countries, 2000 [8]

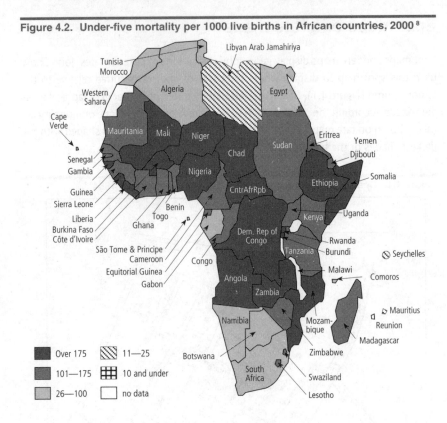

If the bars are horizontal (Figure 2.3), rather than vertical (Figure 3.4), there is likely to be enough space to include clear labels for the categories. In some cases it can also help to arrange the bars according to their length.

Line graphs

Line graphs (Figure 6.1) are best suited for displaying the amount of change or difference in a continuous variable, which is usually shown on the vertical axis. For example, serum cholesterol levels – on the vertical axis – can be plotted over time on the horizontal axis. When reading a line graph, it is important to check the scale of the vertical axis. If a logarithmic scale is used, the interpretation changes from absolute amounts to rates or proportions of change. For this type of graph, scale breaks can be used on the vertical axis, but these should be clearly indicated.

Box 4.3. A word of caution

Although inappropriate, scale breaks are often used and can come in different forms. In fact, they sometimes are used to deliberately exaggerate relationships and this use may only be apparent upon careful examination of the vertical axis. When reading a chart, it is important to examine the vertical axis carefully to make sure that you understand clearly the scale used and that there are no hidden breaks.

Frequency distributions and histograms

A frequency distribution is the organization of a data set into contiguous mutually exclusive intervals so that the number or proportion of observations falling in each interval is apparent. They are often displayed with a histogram, which looks like a bar chart with all the bars stacked together in an orderly fashion, with no space between the bars (Figure 6.7). The heights of the bars represent either the number or percent of observations within each interval. The overall shape of this distribution can be highly informative. Frequency polygons, which are essentially a line that connects the middle of each of the bars of the histogram, are also used extensively. The bell-shaped curve of the normal distribution is one important example (Figure 4.3).

Figure 4.3. The normal distribution curve

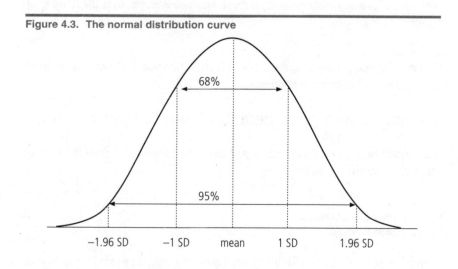

Normal distributions

The normal distribution has extremely useful characteristics. A large number of statistical tests and calculations can be used if the observations follow a normal distribution. It is useful to know that about two-thirds of the values under a normal distribution curve fall within one standard deviation of the mean, and approximately 95% fall within two standard deviations of the mean.

Summary numbers

Means, medians and mode

One set of summary numbers are those that measure central tendency, that is, they attempt to characterize the center of a sample of measurements.

The mean
Most prominent, and often the most appropriate, is the sample average or mean, which for a sample with n values for a variable such as $x_i = $ body weight, would be:

$$mean = \bar{x} = \sum_{i=1}^{n} x_i / n$$

The median
The median is defined as the middle after all the measurements have been put in order according to their values. The median is especially useful when a few values are much larger than others. For this reason, personal income tends to be reported as

median income rather than average income, since the median is not affected unduly by the very high incomes for a very few members of the sample. Note that income for a country is sometimes reported as per capita income. This number can be quite different from median income which is the middle of the distribution of the individual incomes, most of which are likely to represent the income supporting an entire family, whereas per capita income represents these incomes averaged over the number of persons in the country.

The mode
Another important measure is the mode, which is the value of the measurement in the sample that occurs most frequently.

Variances, standard deviations and standard errors

Measures of variability are another group of summary numbers. The three most useful measures of variability are the

- variance
- standard deviation
- standard error.

Each of these is related to how unlike each other the individuals are in a sample of measurements. These measures of variability can be calculated on;

- the differences between members for all possible pairs of measurements in the sample or
- the difference between each observation in the sample and the sample mean, that is $(x_i - \bar{x})^2$: the squared deviation from the mean.

Such calculations, while appealing, are rather cumbersome. An algebraic equivalent is often used. This is a formula for the sample variance – with subscripts dropped for simplicity:

$$s^2 = \frac{\sum x^2 - (\sum)^2/n}{n-1}$$

The numerator of the above equation can also be written as:

$$SS\,(x) - \sum (x = \bar{x})^2 = \sum x^2 - (\sum x)^2/n$$

This term is often called the sum of squared deviations about the mean, or simply the

$$\text{Sum of Squares} = SS(x).$$

Note that the variance is very close to the average of the squared deviations from the mean. The standard deviation is simply the square root of the variance or $s = \sqrt{s^2}$ and the standard error, which is:

$$SE = s_{\bar{x}} = s/\sqrt{n},$$

is typically called the standard error of the mean. The standard error of the mean reflects how unlike each other all possible means of samples of size n might be if each sample were randomly selected from the same population as the initial sample.

Basic concepts of statistical inference

The process of using a sample to make inferences about a population is perhaps the most vital aspect of epidemiologic research. The conceptual underpinnings for statistical inference are based on the process of taking a single random sample of a specific size from a population and using this sample to make judgments about the population as a whole. Typically, these judgments are made in terms of means, variances or other summarizing numbers. Summarizing numbers for the population are called parameters and are represented by Greek letters such as:

- μ = mean,
- σ = standard deviation and
- β = regression coefficient.

Estimates of these parameters obtained from a sample are represented by $\overline{x}$, s and b, respectively.

Using samples to understand populations

Random samples
The process of selecting a sample from a population is essential to statistical inference. The first step is to select a random sample, whereby each member of the population has an equal chance of being selected for the sample (see Chapter 3). There are numerous sampling strategies and texts to help guide this process.
   Example: calculating a sample mean
   10 people are randomly selected from a population and their weights are measured in kilograms as 82.3, 67.3, 68.6, 57.7, 67.3, 60.5, 61.8, 54.5, 73.2 and 85.9 so that

$$\overline{x} = \sum_{i=1}^{n} x_i / n = 67.9 \text{ kg},$$

which is an estimate of μ = population mean weight.

Of course, another random sample selected from this same population and the weights measured for this new group could lead to a different sample mean; say, $\overline{x}$ = 68.2 kg, as an estimate of the same population mean, μ. One of these sample means is not better than the other, but this does raise the question as to the value of an individual sample mean as an estimate of the population mean when it is so easy to take another sample and obtain a different value for $\overline{x}$. To put this into context, the value is derived from the process used to obtain the estimate.
   If this process were repeated a very large number of times, a very long list of sample means could be calculated (Box 4.4). How well a sample mean estimates the population mean can be assessed by examining the characteristics of this long list of

sample means. If the mean of all these sample means, that is the mean of the means, is the same as the population mean, then the sample mean is an unbiased estimate of the population mean. That is, on average, it provides the correct answer.

Confidence intervals

Confidence intervals are one of the most useful tools in epidemiology. In general, a confidence interval uses these concepts to create reasonable bounds for the population mean, based on information from a sample. They are easy to prepare and relatively easy to understand.

Box 4.4. Standard error of the mean

Clearly, it is also preferable that these sample means be very similar to each other, so that any one of them is likely to be close to the true value of the population mean. The standard deviation for this long list of sample means, a measure of how similar these sample means are to each other, is called the **standard error of the mean**. Note that the long list of sample means is not actually needed in order to estimate this standard error, as it can be calculated from a single sample standard deviation as presented in the formula.

Calculating a confidence interval

To construct a confidence interval, a lower bound and an upper bound are calculated. For the sample of weights, with n = 10 and $\bar{x}$ = 67.9, the standard deviation calculated for this sample is s = 10.2 kg. The lower and upper bounds are:

$$Lower\ bound \quad \bar{x} \quad (2.68)s/\sqrt{n} \quad 69.7 \quad 2.68(10.2)/3.16 \quad 61.05$$

$$Upper\ bound \quad \bar{x} \quad (2.68)s/\sqrt{n} \quad 69.7 \quad 2.68(10.2)/3.16 \quad 78.35$$

It may be helpful to write the resulting confidence interval as follows;

$$C(61.05 < \mu < 78.35) = 0.95$$

which clearly indicates that it is a 95% confidence interval for the population mean. The length of this interval is 78.35 − 61.05 = 17.30 kg, which is longer than might be desirable. Note that the shorter the interval the better, and that a larger sample will likely produce a shorter interval. Also note that the sample mean $\bar{x}$ is guaranteed to be within this interval. In fact, in this case, it is exactly in the middle of the interval; whereas the population mean, while likely to be included, is certainly not guaranteed to be within this interval.

Degrees of freedom

Note that the number 2.68 used in these calculations is from the t distribution with n-1 = 9 degrees of freedom. However, if the sample size is above n = 30, then the number 2.00 will be very close to the value in the table. For very large samples, the number will be 1.96. Tables for this distribution are available in most standard statistics texts and online statistics resources.

This example focuses on confidence intervals for μ; however, the concept is broadly used for other parameters, including those from regression analyses and for odds ratios, among many others. The interpretation is similar to that described below for means. Interpreting a confidence interval can sometimes be a bit confusing (Box 4.5).

Box 4.5. Interpreting a confidence interval

It is conceivable that there could be a long list of random samples taken from a population and that a confidence interval could be calculated based on the information from each sample. The result would be a long list of confidence intervals and the expectation is that, if this were done and if α = 0.05, then 95% of them would contain the true value of the population mean within their bounds and 5% would not. Unfortunately, for a specific sample one does not know if the confidence interval obtained from the study sample is one of the 95% or one of the 5%.

Interpreting measures outside the confidence interval

When interpreting confidence intervals, one needs to know what to do with measures that fall outside of the interval. In the example above, the weights range from 61.05 to 78.35 kg. Is it reasonable to believe that the population mean could be 80.0 kg? One would expect that 95% of such confidence intervals would in fact contain the population mean. It seems unlikely that the population mean is $\mu = 80.0$ kg, although it could be, if this interval happens to be one of the 5% rather than one of the 95%. Even though there is some risk in claiming that $\mu \neq 80.0$ kg, the risk is small, and further, it was set to be small when $\alpha = 0.05$ was used to create a 95% confidence interval. It is important to understand that this risk of saying that $\mu \neq 80.0$ (when in fact it is 80.0 kg) is set by the investigator who calculates the confidence interval. Values other than $\alpha = 0.05$ can be used, with $\alpha = 0.01$ being perhaps the other value most commonly used; however $\alpha = 0.05$ is most common and most readily accepted. Figure 5.2. shows an example of a confidence interval.

We can use a confidence interval to test a hypothesis, namely, the hypothesis that $\mu = 80.0$ kg. In this case, the hypothesis was tested and rejected based on the lower and upper limits of the confidence interval. In general, confidence intervals can be used in this way to test hypotheses; however, there is a more formal approach described in Box 4.6.

Hypothesis tests, p-values, statistical power

Hypothesis-testing is relatively straightforward. We need to make a careful statement of the statistical hypothesis to be tested, the p-value associated with this test and the statistical power the test has for "detecting" a difference of a specified magnitude.

The p-value

In the above situation, the null hypothesis was rejected because the observed outcome was deemed to be too unlikely or rare under the assumption that the null hypothesis was true. The cut point for rarity in this circumstance was set when the α-level was set at $\alpha = 0.05$. A more precise measure of the rarity of this observed outcome, again under the assumption that the null hypothesis is true, can be obtained readily. It is simply the area below -3.19 plus the area above +3.19 in a t distribution with 9 degrees of freedom. The area below -3.19 is 0.011, the area above +3.19 is also 0.011 so that the total is $p = 0.022$. This area is called the p-value and it represents the likelihood that a value for the mean of a random sample from this population, would be as far away as 67.9 or farther from $\mu = 80$ kg on either side. That is, the observed outcome is so rare that it is difficult to believe that $\mu = 80$ kg. The p-value and α-level are related in the sense that if $\alpha = 0.05$, then the null hypothesis would be rejected when $p < 0.05$.

Statistical power

In the description of the two-sample t-test below, there is reference to the null hypothesis:

$$H_0 : \mu_1 - \mu_2 = 0, vs$$
$$H_1 : \mu_1 - \mu_2 \neq 0$$

which examines the differences between the means of two populations. If these are two populations of body weights, then, in this context, clearly, the larger the difference between the two population means, the easier it will be to reject this null hypothesis using the sample means.

Box 4.6. Example: testing a hypothesis

Using the example above, with $\overline{x}$ = 69.7kg, and s = 10.2 kg, the formal process can be expressed as:

- *The hypothesis:*

We want to know whether it is reasonable to believe that the population mean could be $\mu = 80$. In order to set up a statistical test for this question, we select two options for comparison:

- the null hypothesis: $H_0: \mu = 80$ *kg* and
- the alternative: $H_1: \mu \neq 80$ *kg.*

Our statistical test is set up to select one of these two. If H_1 is selected, the usual statement is that the null hypothesis H_0 has been rejected. Note that the alternative is expressed as $H_1: \mu \neq 80$ *kg* rather than either $\mu > 80$ or $\mu < 80$. This implies that a two-tailed test is to be done rather than a one-tailed test as would be the case if either of the other two alternatives were used. In general, a two-tailed test should be used for basic epidemiologic applications as the conditions necessary for comfortable use of the one-tailed test in this context are rare.

- *The assumptions.* In this case, the assumptions are that a random sample was selected from a normal distribution. If the sample size is larger than n = 30, a normal distribution is not essential.
- *The α-level:* Use $\alpha = 0.05$ unless there is a compelling reason to do otherwise. The most common other level used is $\alpha = 0.01$.
- *The test statistic:* The test statistic equivalent to the use of the confidence interval above to test this hypothesis is the one-sample t-test as shown in the formula below. This formula uses the same information used to construct the confidence interval but is organized in a different form.

$$t = \frac{\overline{x} - \mu}{s/\sqrt{n}}$$

- *The critical region:* Reject the null hypothesis $H_0: \mu = 80$ *kg* if the value for the test statistic is not between $\pm\, t_{0.975}$ (9) = 2.68. Note that this implies that a region has been delineated by the cutpoints -2.68 and +2.68, with the rejection region being anything below -2.68 or above +2.68.
- *The result:*

$$t = \frac{69.7 - 80}{10.2/\sqrt{10}} = -3.19$$

- *The conclusion:* Since the value calculated for *t* is not between $\pm\, t_{0.975}$ (9) = 2.68, the conclusion is to reject the null hypothesis $H_0: \mu = 80$ *kg* in favor of the alternative $H_1: \mu \neq 80$ *kg.* One interpretation is that the sample mean $\overline{x}$ = 69.7 kg is so far away from $\mu = 80$ *kg* that it is difficult to believe that the true value of the population mean could be 80 kg. That is, the observed outcome with $\overline{x}$ = 69.7, while certainly possible, is simply too unlikely or rare for the mean for a sample taken from a population with $\mu = 80$ *kg.*

An important question deals with the likelihood that the null hypothesis would be rejected if the difference was as large as, say 4.0 kg. That is, what is the likelihood that a difference as large as 4.0 kg would be "detected"? This likelihood is called *statistical power*. Of course, the higher the power the better, provided costs are reasonable. Power is affected by the sample size (larger being better) and the variance of the individual observations (smaller being better). Further, changing a from $a = 0.05$ to $a = 0.01$ reduces the power.

Clearly, when hypotheses are tested, errors can be made. If the null hypothesis is rejected when it is in fact true, then this error is called the a-error, and the likelihood of this error is established when the a-level is set prior to conducting the test. Again, in general, we use $a = 0.05$ unless we have a compelling reason to do otherwise.

On the other side, when the null hypothesis is accepted, an error can also be made and this error is called the β-error. This error is discussed further in the section on sample size. The likelihood that the null hypothesis will be rejected when it should be, is statistical power and has the value, Power = 1-. The possible outcomes for a hypothesis test are:

Test result	The truth	
	H₀ correct	**H₀ wrong**
Accept H₀	OK	*Type II or β-error*
Reject H₀	*Type I or α-error*	OK

Basic methods

The basic methods for epidemiology are:

- t-tests
- chi square tests
- correlation
- regression.

t-tests

It is common in epidemiology to have two samples representing two different populations and to want an answer to the question of whether the two sample means are sufficiently different to lead one to conclude that the two populations they represent have different means. The t-test uses a statistic that, under the null hypothesis, tests whether these two means differ significantly. The t-test, especially its two-sample version can be used for this situation. The hypothesis:

$$H_0 : \mu_1 - \mu_2 = 0, vs$$
$$H_1 : \mu_1 - \mu_2 \neq 0$$

is tested with the use of the t-statistic with ($n_1 + n_2$ -2) degrees of freedom:

$$t = \frac{\bar{x}_1 - \bar{x}_2}{s_p \sqrt{\frac{1}{n_1} + \frac{1}{n_2}}}, \; where \; s_p^2 = \frac{(n_1 - 1)s_1^2 + (n_2 - 1)s_2^2}{(n_1 - 1) + (n_2 - 1)}$$

Chi-squared tests for cross tabulations

Cross tabulations, or contingency tables, are tools for displaying numbers of participants classified according to two or more factors or variables. Table 3.4 is a typical example, with r = 2 rows and c = 2 columns of data for a rxc or 2x2 table. This table displays the association between two exposure and two disease status categories. Close examination of the table leads to the inevitable question of whether or not there is evidence of an association between exposure and disease, that is, to a test of the hypothesis:

H_0: *There is no association between this classification for exposure and this classification for disease status,* versus

H_1: *There is association between this classification for exposure and this classification for disease status.*

For 2x2 tables, this hypothesis can also address comparisons between two proportions. In this case, the proportions of interest are:

P_E = Proportion of those who were **exposed** who developed the disease,

P_{NE} = Proportion of those who were **not exposed** who developed the disease,

so that the hypothesis can be expressed as:

H_0: $P_E = P_{NE}$, versus

H_1: $P_E \neq P_{NE}$.

To test this hypothesis, we compare the *Observed Frequency, O* in each cell to the *Expected Frequency, E* that would be there if the null hypothesis were completely true. *E* can be calculated to create the following table:

$$E = \frac{(Total\ for\ row\ containing\ cell) \times (Total\ for\ column\ containing\ cell)}{Overall\ total\ for\ table}$$

Cell	O	E	O-E	(O-E)²	(O-E)²/E
1	50	34.12	15.88	252.22	7.39
2	11	26.88	-15.88	252.22	9.38
3	16	31.88	-15.88	252.22	7.91
4	41	25.12	15.88	252.22	10.04
Total	118	118	0.00		34.72

The total in the last column is the calculated value for $\chi^2(1)$, which is the notation for the chi-square test statistic with one degree of freedom. In general, the number of degrees of freedom is $df = (r-1) \times (c-1)$. The calculated value, 34.72, is much larger than the value in the chi-square table for $\alpha = 0.05$, which is 3.84; hence we reject the null hypothesis. Tables for the chi-square distribution are available online or in any standard statistical text book (see Chapter 11).

Correlation

In general, correlation quantifies the degree to which two variables vary together (Chapter 5). If two variables are independent, then the value of one has no relationship to the value for the other. If they are correlated, then the value for one is related to the value of the other, either high when the other is high or being high when the other is low. There are several tools available for measuring correlation. The most commonly used is the Pearson Product Moment Correlation Coefficient, calculated as:

Box 4.7. Interpreting the relationship between two variables

It is always useful to examine a picture of the relationship between the two variables with a scatter plot (see Figure 1.1). Plots with groups of dots in more than one location or with dots that seem to fall along a curved line may well imply that the correlation coefficient is not providing a meaningful summary of the relationship between the two variables.

$$r_{xy} = \frac{\sum xy - (\sum x)(\sum y)/n}{\sqrt{[\sum x^2 - (\sum x)^2/n][\sum y^2 - (\sum y)^2/n]}} = \frac{SS(xy)}{\sqrt{SS(x)SS(y)}}$$

This coefficient measures linear association and ranges between $-1 \le r \le 1$. It is near $+1$ when the there is strong positive linear association and is near -1 when there is strong negative association, that is, when a low value for x tends to imply a high one for y. When $r = 0$, there is no linear association. A word of caution is advised (Box 4.7)

Regression

Using and interpreting regression models
Regression models are vital tools for data analysis and are used extensively in epidemiological research. Their underlying concepts are not complex, although the calculations can be. Fortunately, computer programs can take care of the calculations. As such complexity is not needed in this text, our focus is on using and interpreting these models.

Different regression models
Three types of regression models are fundamental to epidemiological research:

- linear regression
- logistic regression
- Cox proportional hazards regression, a type of survival analysis.

Key concept for regression models
To use these models, we assume that variables influence each other. For example, we can consider that body weight is influenced by factors such as age or gender. The value of interest is the dependent variable (e.g. body weight) and the identifiable factors are independent variables. It is the nature of the dependent variable that most distinguishes the three models from each other.

- *Linear regression models.*
  the dependent variable needs to be a continuous variable with its frequency distribution being the normal distribution.

- *Logistic regression models.*
  the dependent variable is derived from the presence or absence of a characteristic, typically represented by 0 or 1.
- *Cox proportional hazards models:*
  the dependent variable represents the time from a baseline of some type to the occurrence of an event of interest.

Survival analysis – as done with Cox proportional hazards models – has an additional complexity in that censoring status needs to be considered as well.

Linear regression

We can use the linear regression tool to address a broad set of issues, ranging from standard Analysis of Variance (ANOVA), to simple linear regression, and multiple linear regression. In all these cases, the dependent variable is a continuous measure (such as body weight), and the independent variables may be both continuous and categorical.

Dependent variable

A typical model, representing the dependent variable Y and k independent variables, might look like:

$$Y = \beta_0 + \beta_1 x_1 + \beta_2 x_2 + \cdots + \beta_k x_k + \varepsilon,$$

where:

Y = Dependent variable, (e.g. body weight)
β_0 = Intercept or scaling factor
β_i = Coefficient for the independent variable x_i
x_i = Value for independent variable x_i
ε = Value for what is not accounted for by the other factors

The term $\beta_i x_i$ represents the portion of the dependent variable, Y = body weight, associated with, or attributed to, the independent variable; say, x_i = age. Also, the term ε represents what is left over after the other terms have been taken into account and is sometimes referred to as the "error term."

By this process, we can consider that the body weight for an individual is made up of pieces, with one piece for each of the factors being represented by the independent variables, plus two other pieces – these being the intercept or scaling factor β_0 and whatever is left over – represented by ε. Clearly, the less that is left over, the better, in the sense that the model is "explaining" more. We can quantify the usefulness of a specific regression model by calculating the proportion of the total variation of the dependent variable that is accounted for by the regression equation:

$$R^2 = \frac{SS(Model)}{SS(Y)}.$$

Independent variables

If the independent variable is a continuous variable such as x_i = age, then the interpretation of β_i is straightforward and represents the incremental change in the dependent variable, Y = body weight, associated with a unit change in x_i = age, adjusted for all other terms in the model. This is very much like the slope term in simple linear regression, so if β_{Age} = 2.0 kg, our interpretation is that the estimated body weight goes up 2.0 kg for each one year increment in age, adjusted for all the other terms in the model.

The situation for independent variables that represent categories is a bit different and needs careful attention. A typical example is a variable indicating sex, for which the values could be set at x_1 = 1 if male and x_1 = 0 if female. In this case, the category for which the value is x_1 = 0 is often called the reference group, to which we will compare the category x_1 = 1. For linear regression models, the coefficient for this term is:

$$\beta_1 = \mu_{males} - \mu_{females}$$

that is, the difference between the mean weight, males – females, adjusted for all the other terms in the model.

Multiple variables

When we have three or more categories, the situation is slightly more complex; however, this is common and the correct interpretation is important. An example is blood type with the three categories A, B, and O. For this situation, we need two independent variables – one less than the number of categories. Their values are:

Blood type	x_1	x_2
A	1	0
B	0	1
O	0	0

In this case, the referent group is the "O" category, and

$$\beta_1 = \mu_A - \mu_O$$
$$\beta_2 = \mu_B - \mu_O$$

Here, β_1 is the difference between the mean values for A – O, adjusted for all the terms in the model. With this formula, we can compare A and O directly, and B and O directly, but not A and B. We would have to assign different values to x_1 and x_2 in order to compare A to B.

The formulation above refers to population values for which estimates would be obtained by fitting such a model to a specific set of data. The first step is to test the hypothesis concerning the full set of βs collectively, that is to test:

$$H_0 : \beta_1 = \beta_2 = \cdots = \beta_k = 0 ,$$

If this hypothesis is rejected so that there is evidence that at least one of the βs can be considered to be non-zero, then it is reasonable to progress with the testing of the coefficients for the individual terms. If none can be considered to be non-zero, then the model as stated has no meaningful terms and therefore has little value.

Logistic regression

In the example above, the value for the dependent variable was body weight, a continuous measurement. We may also be interested in factors associated with the presence or absence of obesity, defined perhaps as having a BMI ≥ 30. Logistic regression is a powerful and flexible analytical tool for such situations. Our outcome of interest is typically an odds ratio comparing the odds, (for example, of obesity for males versus females), adjusted for a collection of other factors.

The logistic regression model, as shown below, is ideal for this purpose. The regression model is based on the dependent variable ln(odds) where ln represents the natural logarithmic scale (base e) and odds are defined as the likelihood p of the event occurring divided by the likelihood of it not occurring, $1 - p$, sometimes listed as

$$odds = p\,/(1-p)\,,$$

So the model becomes

$$\ln(odds) = \beta_0 + \beta_1 x_1 + \beta_2 x_2 + \cdots + \beta_k x_k + \varepsilon$$

or equivalently,

$$odds = e^{\beta_0 + \beta_1 x_1 + \beta_2 x_2 + \cdots + \beta_k x_k + \varepsilon}$$

where the x_i are defined as they were for the linear regression model above. To interpret the coefficients for these models, we need to focus on odds and odds ratios rather than means, as was the case for linear regression. For example, for the independent variable, x_1 = gender, with $x_1 = 1$ for males and $x_1 = 0$ for females, then the coefficient β_1 is used in the equation:

$$e^{\beta_1} = OR_{males/females}$$

and the term is interpreted as the obesity odds ratio for males versus females, adjusted for the other terms in the model. The term e^{β_1}, obtained from analyzing the data, is an estimate of this odds ratio.

For the independent variable x_2 = age, measured in years, the term has an interpretation similar to that for the slope in linear regression, this being

$$e^{\beta_2} = OR_{per\ year\ increment}$$

If the adjusted $OR_{per\ year\ increment} = 1.2$, then the odds for obesity are 20% higher for each one year increment in age, adjusted for the other terms in the model.

If $OR_{per\ year\ increment} = 0.75$, then the odds for obesity for a one year increment in age are 75% of those for the previous year, adjusted for the other terms in the model.

Survival analyses and Cox proportional hazards models

For many situations, we are interested in the time until an event occurs (see Figure 8.4). For the obesity situation above, suppose that a group of patients had been successfully treated for obesity and they were being followed post-treatment to assess factors that are associated with obesity reoccurrence. In this case, we would be interested in measuring the time from the end of the initial treatment until obesity reoccurrence.

The Cox proportional hazards model is an appropriate regression model for such situations. The dependent variable represents time until obesity reoccurrence. The independent variables can be the same as for the logistic regression example and the regression equation is:

$$h(t) = h_0(t)e^{\,\beta_1 x_1 + \beta_2 x_2 + \cdots + \beta_k x_k}$$

where
h(t) = hazard of the event, having "survived" until time t without an event,
$h_0(t)$ = baseline hazard rate.
Note that there is no β_0 to serve as an intercept or scaling factor as this is the role of the baseline hazard rate $h_0(t)$.

The only complicating issue for this model is that we need to account for censoring (Box 4.10).

This term is interpreted as the obesity relative risk for males versus females, adjusted for the other terms in the model. The term e^{β_1}, obtained from analysing the data, is an estimate of this relative risk.

For the independent variable x_2 = age, measured in years, the term has an interpretation similar to that for the slope in linear regression, this being

$$e^{\beta_2} = RR_{\text{per year increment}}$$

The interpretation is similar to that for odds ratios in this example for logistic regression.

Box 4.10. Censoring

Censoring is a process for dealing with follow-up time, when the event of interest doesn't happen during the overall follow-up period. This is typically due to drop-out or other reasons for loss to follow-up, but it may also be due to some of the participants "surviving" the complete follow-up time without the event occurring. The follow-up time for an individual participant is said to be censored at, say 15 months, if the person was event-free for 15 months and then was either lost to follow-up or the study ended at that point.

Otherwise, this model is used much like logistic re-gression, except that it provides estimates for hazard ratios or relative risk rather than for odds ratios. That is, for the independent variable, x_1 = gender, with $x_1 = 1$ for males and $x_1 = 0$ for females, then the coefficient β_1 is used in the equation:

$$e^{\beta_1} = RR_{\text{males}/\text{females}}$$

Kaplan-Meier survival curves

Kaplan-Meier survival curves are commonly used to display survival data (see Figure 8.4). They can be used to display any type of time-to-event data. If the event that we are recording is death, then we use the vertical axis to show the proportion alive at a specific point in time, and put time on the horizontal axis. These proportions range from 1.0 at the outset down to 0.0, if all members of the group die during follow-up. Kaplan-Meier curves are clear and easy to interpret and relatively easy to make. The only complication is dealing with the censoring, as discussed above.

Kaplan and Meier solved this problem, which is why these curves carry their name. Their solution was to plot the curves with survival time on the horizontal axis rather than calendar time. Then, using follow-up time as a reference, they assumed that the individual who was censored at 15 months survived until the next event, in follow-up time, occurred. That is, they allowed the individual to "live" a little longer, but only as long as the next person to "die."

Sample size issues

One of the problems we often have in epidemiological investigations is figuring out how large a sample we need to answer a specific question. Our sample size must be big enough for the study to have appropriate statistical power – the ability to demonstrate an association if one exists (see Chapter 3). We base sample size calculations on a number of study design factors:

- prevalence
- acceptable error
- the detectable difference.

There are numerous formulae and computer programs that simplify the task considerably. Two helpful and relatively simple formulae are:

- the two sample t-test and
- the test comparing two proportions.

Two sample t-test

For the two sample t-test, the formula is, for $\alpha = 0.05$,

$$N = n_1 + n_2 = \frac{4\sigma^2 (z_{0.975} + z_{1-\beta})^2}{(d = \mu_1 - \mu_2)^2}.$$

This formula requires that we specify the population variance σ^2, the values from the normal distribution for $z_{0.975}=1.96$, $z_{1-\beta}$, and d = difference that we want to detect. The term $z_{1-\beta}$ represents the desired statistical power. A desirable level for power is $1-\beta = 0.80$. Hence, for the example of body weights, $\sigma^2 = 64$ kg is reasonable, $z_{0.975} = 1.96$, and $z_{0.80} = 0.842$ so that if we want to reject the null hypothesis of no difference between the means of the two populations when the difference between these two means is 4 kg or more, the number needed for both samples combined is:

$$N = n_1 + n_2 = \frac{4\sigma^2 (z_{0.975} + z_{1-\beta})^2}{(d = \mu_1 - \mu_2)^2} = \frac{4(64)(1.96 + 0.842)^2}{4^2} = 125.62$$

It is common that values for σ^2 are not available. Sometimes reasonable numbers can be obtained from other studies; however, it is prudent to calculate more than one value for *N*, by using different combinations of values for σ^2 and, d, and for different power levels. It is important to note that for values of power, $1-\beta > 0.80$, the gain in power for increases in sample size can be relatively small.

Test comparing proportions

For the test comparing proportions, the situation is very similar except that the formulae is, for $\alpha = 0.05$:

$$N = n_1 + n_2 = \frac{4(Z_{0.975} + Z_{1-\beta})^2 \left[\left(\dfrac{P_1 + P_2}{2}\right)\left(1 - \dfrac{P_1 + P_2}{2}\right)\right]}{(d = P_1 - P_2)^2}$$

Note here that the population proportions P_1 and P_2 must be specified. Hence, to detect the difference between $P_1 = 0.60$ and $P_2 = 0.70$, with $\alpha = 0.05$, power = $1-\beta = 0.80$, the calculation is:

$$N = n_1 + n_2 = \frac{4(1.96 - 0.842)^2 \left[\left(\dfrac{0.60 + 0.70}{2}\right)\left(1 - \dfrac{0.60 + 0.70}{2}\right)\right]}{(d = 0.10)^2} = 714.46.$$

For this situation as well, it is prudent to complete this calculation several times, varying the lever for power and the values of P_1 and P_2.

Meta-analysis

Meta-analysis is defined as the statistical synthesis of the data from separate but similar (comparable) studies, leading to a quantifiable summary of the pooled results to identify the overall trend (see Chapter 5). An example is shown in Figure 5.8.

Meta-analysis differs from most medical and epidemiological studies in that no new data are collected. Instead, results from previous studies are combined. Steps in carrying out meta-analysis include:

- formulating the problem and study design;
- identifying relevant studies;
- excluding poorly conducted studies or those with major methodological flaws; and
- measuring, combining and interpreting the results.

Which studies are identified and whether they are included or excluded from the meta-analysis are crucial factors. Another important step is measuring the results of the studies on a single scale. This allows comparisons to be made between studies even if they used different measures of outcome. Meta-analysis is a relatively new scientific method; research into the best techniques to use is still ongoing and expanding into new areas. It is not yet as well-accepted as other statistical techniques that have a longer tradition of use.

The use of meta-analysis in medicine and epidemiology has increased in recent years for ethical reasons, cost issues, and the need to have an overall idea of effects of a particular intervention in different population groups. This is particularly true in the area of clinical trials, where the sample size of individual trials is often too small to permit conclusions to be drawn from any one trial, although conclusions can be drawn from aggregated results. For example, meta-analysis showed that aspirin has a significant effect in preventing a second heart attack or stroke, even though no single study had convincingly shown this. These issues are taken up in greater detail in the next chapter on causation.

Study questions

1. Calculate the mean, median, variance, standard deviation and standard error for the sample of n = 10 body weights given in this chapter.
2. Why is personal income often reported as median income rather than average income?
3. What are the major differences among linear regression, logistic regression and regression models for survival analyses?
4. What is more preferable, a wide confidence interval or a narrow one and why?
5. What information should the title for a table presenting data or results contain?
6. What is the interpretation of the coefficient $b_1 = 5.0$ for the independent variable gender, with $x_1 = 1$ for males and $x_1 = 0$ for females when it is obtained from a multiple regression model with y = body weight (kg) as the dependent variable?
7. What is the interpretation of the coefficient $b1 = 0.5$ for the independent variable x = age (years), when it is obtained from a multiple regression model with y = body weight (kg) as the dependent variable?

References

1. Hosmer DW, Lemeshow S. *Applied Logistic Regression* 2nd ed. John Wiley & Sons Inc., New York, 2000.
2. Hosmer DW, Lemeshow S. *Applied Survival Analyses: Regression Modeling of Time to Event Data.* John Wiley & Sons Inc., New York, 1999.
3. Petitti DB. *Meta-Analysis, Decision Analysis and Cost-Effectiveness Analysis: Methods for Quantitative Synthesis in Medicine.* New York, Oxford University Press, 1994.
4. Whitehead A. *Meta-Analysis of Controlled Clinical Trials.* Chichester, John Wiley & Sons Ltd., 2002.
5. Draper NR, Smith H. *Applied Regression Analyses* 3rd ed. New York, John Wiley & Sons Inc, 1998.
6. Gilbert EW. Pioneer maps of health and disease in England. *Geog J* 1958;124:172-183.
7. Tufte ER. *The visual display of quantitative information.* Cheshire, Graphics Press, 1983.
8. Gordon B, Mackay R, Rehfuess E. *Inheriting the world: the atlas of children's health and the environment.* Geneva, World Health Organization, 2004.

Chapter 5
Causation in epidemiology

Key messages

- The study of causation of diseases and injuries is fundamental to epidemiology.
- There is seldom one single cause of a specific health outcome.
- Causal factors can be arranged into a hierarchy from the most proximal to the distal socio-economic factors.
- Criteria for judging the evidence of causality include: temporal relationship, plausibility, consistency, strength, dose–response relationship, reversibility and study design.

A major focus of epidemiology is informing efforts to prevent and control disease and promote health. To do this, we need to know the causes of disease or injury and the ways in which these causes can be modified. This chapter describes the epidemiological approach to causation.

The concept of cause

An understanding of the causes of disease or injury is important not only for prevention, but also for correct diagnosis and treatment. The concept of cause is the source of much controversy in epidemiology. The process by which we make causal inferences – judgments linking postulated causes and their outcomes – is a major theme of the general philosophy of science, and the concept of cause has different meanings in different contexts.

Sufficient or necessary

A cause of a disease or injury is an event, condition, characteristic or a combination of these factors which plays an important role in producing the health outcome. Logically, a cause must precede an outcome. A cause is termed sufficient when it inevitably produces or initiates an outcome and is termed *necessary* if an outcome cannot develop in its absence. Some diseases are caused completely by genetic factors in the individual, and other causes of a disease interact with genetic factors in making certain individuals more vulnerable than others. The term environmental causes is often used to distinguish these other causes from the genetic causes. It has been pointed out[1] that there are nearly always some genetic and some environmental component causes in every causal mechanism.

Multiple factors

A sufficient cause is not usually a single factor, but often comprises several components (multi-factorial causation). In general, it is not necessary to identify all the components of a sufficient cause before effective prevention can take place, since the removal of one component may interfere with the action of the others and thus prevent the disease or injury. For example, cigarette smoking is one component of the sufficient cause of lung cancer. Smoking is not sufficient in itself to produce the disease: some people smoke for 50 years without developing lung cancer. Other factors, mostly unknown, are involved and genetic factors may play a role. However, the cessation of smoking reduces the number of cases of lung cancer greatly in a population even if the other component causes are not altered (Figure 1.2).

Attributable fraction

The attributable fraction (see chapter 2) can be used to quantify the likely preventive impact of eliminating a specific causal factor. For instance, Table 1.2 shows what would be expected if the smoking asbestos workers had either never smoked or never been exposed to asbestos: never smoking would have decreased the lung cancer death rate from 602 per 100 000 to 58 per 100 000 (a 90% reduction) and never exposed to asbestos, but still smoking, would have reduced the rate from 602 to 123 per 100 000 (an 80% reduction). (Study question 5.3 will explore this further.)

Sufficient and necessary

Each sufficient cause has a necessary cause as a component. For example, in a study of an outbreak of foodborne infection, it may be found that chicken salad and creamy dessert were both sufficient causes of salmonella diarrhoea. However, the ingestion of *Salmonella* bacteria is a necessary cause of this disease. Similarly, there are different components in the causation of tuberculosis, but the infection with *Mycobacterium tuberculosis* is a necessary cause (Figure 5.1). However, a causal factor on its own is often neither necessary nor sufficient, such as tobacco use as a factor for cerebrovascular disease.

The usual approach in epidemiology is to begin with a disease and search for its causes, although it is also possible to start with a potential cause (such as air pollution) and search for its effects. Epidemiology encompasses a whole set of relationships. For example, social class is associated with a range of health problems. Low social class, as measured by income, education, housing and occupation, leads to a general susceptibility to poor health, rather than to a specific effect.[2] A gamut of specific causes of disease could explain why poor people have poor health, among them excessive exposure to infectious agents due to overcrowding, lack of clean water and sanitation, insufficient and unsafe food, and dangerous working conditions. In addition, being at the bottom of the social ladder is in itself associated with poorer health even after taking all the other factors into account.[3] One example of a strong relationship between socioeconomic status and disease is shown in Figure 5.2.[4]

Figure 5.1. Causes of tuberculosis

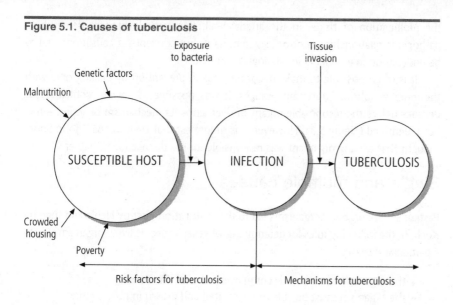

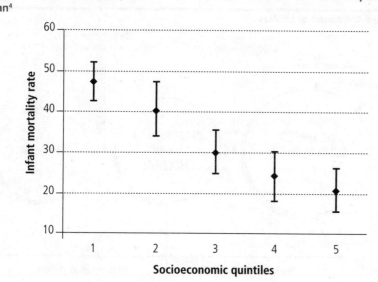

A causal pathway

Epidemiologists have been criticized, particularly by laboratory scientists, for not using the concept of cause in the sense of being the sole requirement for the production of disease. Such a restrictive view of causation, does not take into account the fact that diseases commonly have multiple causes. Prevention strategies often need to be directed simultaneously at more than one factor. In addition, causes can be linked to a *causal pathway* where one factor leads to another until eventually the specific pathogenic agent becomes present in the organ that gets damaged; this can also be called a *hierarchy of causes*. Laboratory scientists might, for example, suggest that the basic cause of coronary heart disease relates to cellular mechanisms involved in

Figure 5.2. Infant mortality rate and socioeconomic status in Islamic Republic of Iran[4]

the proliferation of tissue in the arterial wall. Research directed at determining pathogenic relationships is obviously important, but concepts of causation need to be understood in a wider epidemiological context.

It is often possible to make major progress in prevention by dealing only with the more remote or "upstream" causes. It was possible to prevent cholera cases decades before the responsible organism – let alone its mechanism of action – had been identified (Figure 5.3). However, it is of interest that even in 1854, John Snow thought that a living organism was responsible for the disease (see Chapter 9).

Single and multiple causes

Pasteur's work on microorganisms led to the formulation, first by Henle and then by Koch, of the following rules for determining whether a specific living organism causes a particular disease:

- the organism must be present in every case of the disease;
- the organism must be able to be isolated and grown in pure culture;
- the organism must, when inoculated into a susceptible animal, cause the specific disease;
- the organism must then be recovered from the animal and identified.

Anthrax was the first disease demonstrated to meet these rules, which have since proved useful with many other infectious diseases and with chemical poisoning.

However, for many diseases, both communicable and non-communicable, Koch's rules for determining causation are inadequate. Many causes act together, and a single factor – such as tobacco use – may be a cause of many diseases. In addition, the causative organism may disappear when a disease has developed, making it impossible to demonstrate the organism in the sick person. Koch's postulates are of most value when the specific cause is a highly pathogenic infectious agent, chemical poison or other specific factor, and there are no healthy carriers: a relatively uncommon occurrence.

Figure 5.3. Causes of cholera

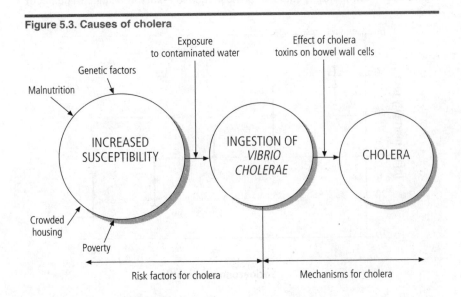

Factors in causation

Four types of factors play a part in the causation of disease, all may be necessary but they are rarely sufficient to cause a particular disease or state:

- *Predisposing factors,* such as age, sex, or specific genetic traits that may result in a poorly functioning immune system or slow metabolism of a toxic chemical. Previous illness may also create a state of susceptibility to a disease agent.
- *Enabling (or disabling) factors* such as low income, poor nutrition, bad housing and inadequate medical care may favour the development of disease. Conversely, circumstances that assist in recovery from illness or in the maintenance of good health could also be called enabling factors. The social and economic determinants of health are just as important as the precipitating factors in designing prevention approaches.
- *Precipitating factors* such as exposure to a specific disease agent may be associated with the onset of a disease.
- *Reinforcing factors* such as repeated exposure, environmental conditions and unduly hard work may aggravate an established disease or injury.

The term "risk factor" is commonly used to describe factors that are positively associated with the risk of development of a disease but that are not sufficient to cause the disease. The concept has proved useful in several practical prevention programmes. Some risk factors (such as tobacco smoking) are associated with several diseases, and some diseases (such as coronary heart disease) are associated with several risk factors (Figure 5.4).

Figure 5.4. Risk factors common to major noncommunicable diseases[5]

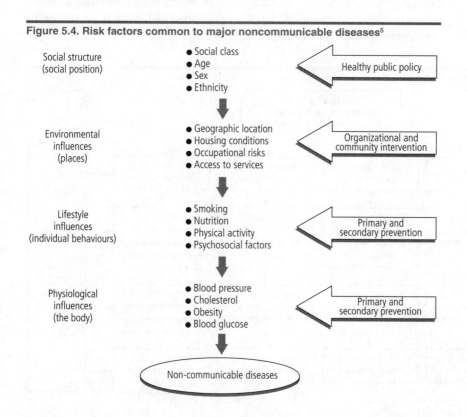

Epidemiological studies can measure the relative contribution of each factor to disease occurrence, and the corresponding potential reduction in disease from the elimination of each risk factor. However, multi-causality means that the sum of the attributable fractions for each risk factor may be greater than 100%.

Interaction

The effect of two or more causes acting together is often greater than would be expected on the basis of summing the individual effects. This phenomenon, called interaction, is illustrated by the particularly high risk of lung cancer in people who both smoke and are exposed to asbestos dust (Table 1.2). The risk of lung cancer in this group is much higher than would be indicated by a simple addition of the risks from smoking (ten times) and exposure to asbestos dust (five times); the risk is multiplied fifty times.

A hierarchy of causes

Multiple causes and risk factors can often be displayed in the form of a hierarchy of causes, where some are the proximal or most immediate causes (precipitating factors) and others are distal or indirect causes (enabling factors). Inhaled tobacco smoke is a proximal cause of lung cancer, while low socio-economic status is a distal cause that is associated with smoking habits and indirectly with lung cancer. Various frameworks have been devised for visualizing the relationships between the distal and proximal causes and the eventual health effects. One such multi-layer framework, DPSEEA (driving forces, pressure, state, exposure, effect, action), was used by WHO to analyse different elements of causation, prevention and indicators in relation to environmental health hazards (Figure 5.5).

Figure 5.5. The DPSEEA framework[6]

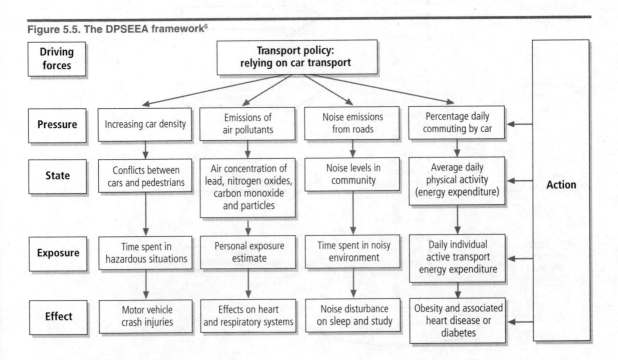

A similar framework was developed for the WHO Global Burden of Disease project.[7] The Multiple Exposures, Multiple Effects framework emphasizes the complex relationships between environmental exposures and child health outcomes. This model takes into account that individual exposures can lead to many different health outcomes, and specific health outcomes can be attributed to many different exposures.[8]

In epidemiological studies linking one or more causes to a health outcome, it is important to consider to what extent different causes are at the same or different levels in the hierarchy. If a "cause of a cause" is included in the analysis together with the cause itself, the statistical method of analysis has to take this into account. The identification of the hierarchy of causes and the quantitative relationships between them will provide one way of describing the mechanism of causation. For example, low socio-economic status is associated in many industrialized nations with more tobacco smoking, which is associated with higher blood pressure, which in turn increases the risk of stroke.

Establishing the cause of a disease

Causal inference is the term used for the process of determining whether observed associations are likely to be causal; the use of guidelines and the making of judgements are involved. The process of judging causation can be difficult and contentious. It has been argued that causal inference should be restricted to the measurement of an effect, rather than as a criterion-guided process for deciding whether an effect is present or not.[1,9] Before an association is assessed for the possibility that it is causal, other explanations, such as chance, bias and confounding, have to be excluded. How these factors are assessed has been described in Chapter 3. The steps in assessing the nature of the relationship between a possible cause and an outcome are shown in Figure 5.6.

Considering causation

A systematic approach to determining the nature of an association was used by the United States Surgeon General to establish that cigarette smoking caused lung cancer.[10] This approach was further elaborated by Hill.[11] On the basis of these concepts, a set of "considerations for causation," listed in the sequence of testing that the epidemiologist should follow to reach a conclusion about a cause of disease, is shown in Table 5.1.

Temporal relationship

The temporal relationship is crucial—the cause must precede the effect. This is usually self-evident, although difficulties may arise in case-control and cross-sectional studies when measurements of the possible cause and effect are made at the same time. In cases where the cause is an exposure that can be at different levels, it is essential that a high enough level be reached before the disease occurs for the correct temporal

Figure 5.6. Assessing the relationship between a possible cause and an outcome

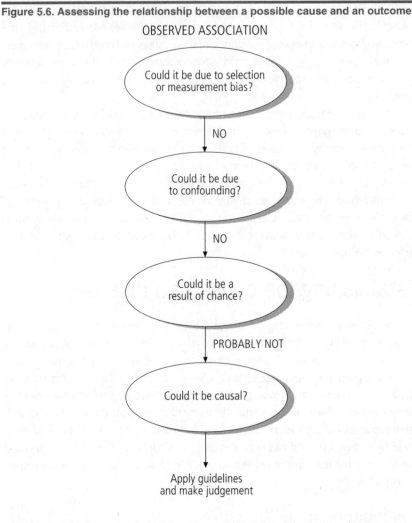

OBSERVED ASSOCIATION

Could it be due to selection
or measurement bias?

NO

Could it be due
to confounding?

NO

Could it be a
result of chance?

PROBABLY NOT

Could it be causal?

Apply guidelines
and make judgement

relationship to exist. Repeated measurement of the exposure at more than one point in time and in different locations may strengthen the evidence.

Table 5.1. Considerations for causation

Temporal relation	Does the cause precede the effect? (essential)
Plausibility	Is the association consistent with other knowledge? (mechanism of action; evidence from experimental animals)
Consistency	Have similar results been shown in other studies?
Strength	What is the strength of the association between the cause and the effect? (relative risk)
Dose–response relationship	Is increased exposure to the possible cause associated with increased effect?
Reversibility	Does the removal of a possible cause lead to reduction of disease risk?
Study design	Is the evidence based on a strong study design?
Judging the evidence	How many lines of evidence lead to the conclusion?

Figure 3.3 is an example of a time series of measurements of exposure and effect. It illustrates high daily temperatures (above 30 °C) in Paris during a two-week period

in August 2003 and the increase of daily mortality during this period. This relationship between heat waves and increased urban mortality has been documented previously in several other cities and is expected to occur with increased frequency as a result of global climate change.[12]

Plausibility

An association is plausible, and thus more likely to be causal, if consistent with other knowledge. For instance, laboratory experiments may have shown how exposure to the particular factor could lead to changes associated with the effect measured. However, biological plausibility is a relative concept, and seemingly implausible associations may eventually be shown to be causal. For example, the predominant view on the cause of cholera in the 1830s involved "miasma" rather than contagion. Contagion was not supported by evidence until Snow's work was published; much later, Pasteur and his colleagues identified the causative agent. Lack of plausibility may simply reflect lack of scientific knowledge. Doubts about the therapeutic effects of acupuncture and homeopathy may be partly attributable to the absence of information about a plausible biological mechanism. A recent example of plausibility being the main reason for a conclusion about causality is variant Creutzfeldt–Jakob disease (vCJD). (Box 5.1)

The study of the health consequences of low-level lead exposure is another example of the initial difficulties in getting conclusive epidemiological evidence, even when animal experiments indicate an effect of lead on the central nervous system. Similar effects in an epidemiological study of children are therefore plausible but, because of potential confounding factors and measurement difficulties, epidemiological studies originally showed conflicting results. However, assessment of all the available epidemiological data leads to the conclusion that children are affected at a low level of exposure to lead[14] (Box 5.2).

Consistency

Consistency is demonstrated by several studies giving the same result. This is particularly important when a variety of designs are used in different settings, since the likelihood that all studies are making the same mistake is thereby minimized. However, a lack of consistency does not exclude a causal association, because different exposure levels and other conditions may reduce the impact of

---

Box 5.1. BSE and vCJD

Variant Creutzfeldt–Jakob disease (vCJD) is the human form of "mad cow disease" or bovine spongiform encephalopathy (BSE). There was an epidemic of BSE in the United Kingdom in 1987.[13] Both diseases are invariably fatal and there are similar pathological changes in the brains of humans with vCJD and cows with BSE. These diseases are examples of transmissible spongiform encephalopathies, which are caused by an infectious agent called a prion. The epidemic in cattle had been caused by feed contaminated with infected carcasses of other cattle, and was finally controlled by banning the use of ruminant proteins as cattle feed. In 1995 there were three cases of vCJD in young people, and by 2002 a total of 139 human cases had been reported. Despite definitive evidence for an oral route of transmission, many experts concluded that the human epidemic was related to the bovine epidemic and caused by the same infective agent. Concerns about human transmission led to changes in blood donation policies and greater use of disposable surgical instruments.

Box 5.2. Lead exposure in children

In the United States of America, regular monitoring of lead exposure in hundreds of thousands of children's blood samples has shown that, while average levels are decreasing since lead was banned from motor-fuels, many children still have elevated levels.[15] The blood lead level at which a risk for damage to the child's brain is considered to occur has been reduced from 250 ug/l in 1995 to 100 ug/l in recent years, and some research indicates that there is a risk at even lower levels.[16] It is plausible that with more precise measurement tools, it may be found that some children are affected at still lower levels. Most of the research on this lingering environmental health problem has been carried out in high-income countries, but increasingly lead exposures and health effects are being reported from low- and middle-income countries.[17]

the causal factor in certain studies. Furthermore, when the results of several studies are being interpreted, the best-designed ones should be given the greatest weight.

Techniques are available for pooling the results of several studies that have examined the same issue, particularly randomized controlled trials. This technique is called meta-analysis (see Chapter 4), and is used to combine the results of several trials, each of which may deal with a relatively small sample, to obtain a better overall estimate of effect (Figure 5.7).[18]

Systematic review uses standardized methods to select and review all relevant studies on a particular topic with a view to eliminating bias in critical appraisal and synthesis. Systematic review as part of the Cochrane Collaboration is sometimes, but not always, coupled with meta-analysis.[19] Figure 5.7 illustrates the results of 113 case-control studies and two cohort studies on the relationship between oral clefts in babies and tobacco use among women who smoked during pregnancy. One important reason for the apparent inconsistency of the results is that several of the early studies were based on small samples. The estimated relative risk in each study is marked by a box; the horizontal lines indicate the 95% confidence intervals. For the aggregated data from all the trials, covering a large number of events, the 95% confidence interval is very narrow. Overall, maternal smoking appears to be associated with a 22% increase in cleft palates: the 95% confidence interval shows that the increase could be at least 10% and as much as 35%.[20]

Figure 5.7. Meta-analysis of the relative risk of cleft palate in the offspring of mothers who smoked during pregnancy compared with the offspring of mothers who did not smoke[20]

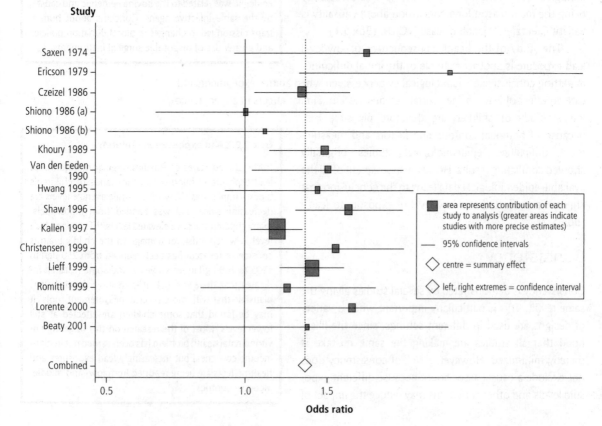

Meta-analysis can also be used to pool results from other types of epidemiological studies such as time-series studies of daily air pollution (particulate matter) and total mortality (Box 5.3).

Strength

A strong association between possible cause and effect, as measured by the size of the risk ratio (relative risk), is more likely to be causal than is a weak association, which could be influenced by confounding or bias. Relative risks greater than 2 can be considered strong. For example, cigarette smokers have a twofold increase in the risk of acute myocardial infarction compared with non-smokers. The risk of lung cancer in smokers, compared with non-smokers, has been shown in various studies to be increased between fourfold and twentyfold. However, associations of such magnitude are rare in epidemiology.

The fact that an association is weak does not preclude it from being causal; the strength of an association depends on the relative prevalence of other possible causes. For example, weak associations have been found between diet and risk of coronary heart disease in observational studies; and although experimental studies on selected populations have been done, no conclusive results have been published. Despite this lack of evidence, diet is generally thought to be a major causative factor in the high rate of coronary heart disease in many industrialized countries.

The probable reason for the difficulty in identifying diet as a risk factor for coronary heart disease is that diets in populations are rather homogeneous and variation over time for one individual is greater than that between people. If everyone has more or less the same diet, it is not possible to identify diet as a risk factor. Consequently, ecological evidence gains importance. This situation has been characterized as one of sick individuals and sick population,[23] meaning that in many high-income countries, whole populations are at risk from an adverse factor.

Dose–response relationship

A dose–response relationship occurs when changes in the level of a possible cause are associated with changes in the prevalence or incidence of the effect. Table 5.2 illustrates the dose–response relationship between noise and hearing loss: the prevalence of hearing loss increases with noise level and exposure time.

The demonstration of such a clear dose–response relationship in unbiased studies provides strong evidence for a causal relationship between exposure and disease.

> **Box 5.3. Air pollution and total mortality**
>
> The results of a large number of time-series studies in different cities in the USA were combined; although some of the studies had conflicting results, a statistically significant association between the exposure and effect was observed.[21] This strengthens the impression that particulate matter air pollution is causing increased mortality, even though the exact mechanism is unclear. A similar meta-analysis of ozone levels and mortality also suggested a causal relationship, but the analysis was limited by "publication bias"[22], meaning that studies which did not achieve statistical significance, or the desired effect, were not published.

Table 5.2. Percentage of people with hearing loss relative to workplace noise exposure[24]

Average noise level during 8-hours (decibels)	Exposure time (years)		
	5	10	40
< 80	0	0	0
85	1	3	10
90	4	10	21
95	7	17	29
100	12	29	41
105	18	42	54
110	26	55	62
115	36	71	64

Figure 5.8. Continuous associations between blood pressure, fruit and vegetable consumption, and heart disease[25]

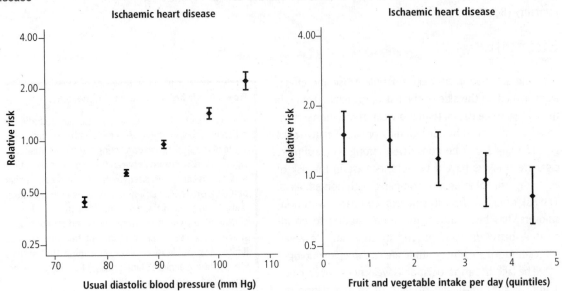

The dose–response relationship shown for fruit and vegetable consumption and relative risk of ischaemic heart disease, inverse to that shown for blood pressure in Figure 5.8, is an example of how socioeconomic circumstances can contribute to health outcomes. Surveys done in the United Kingdom have shown a strong relationship between income level and consumption of fruit and vegetables. Figure 5.9 shows a continuous increase of average fruit and vegetable consumption with increase of income. The figure also shows that people in the lower income deciles spend a greater share of their income on food. The higher cost of diets that have higher proportions of fruit and vegetables may be a factor in this consumption pattern. These relationships are contributing to the broader "dose-response relationship" between income and mortality: the lower the income, the higher the mortality.

Figure 5.9. Fruit and vegetable consumption and socio-economic status[26]

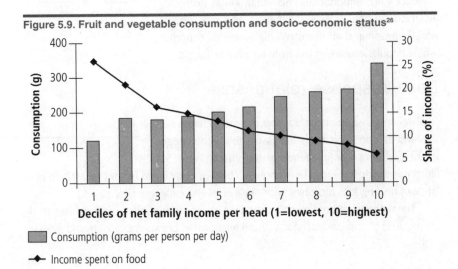

Reversibility

When the removal of a possible cause results in a reduced disease risk, there is a greater likelihood that the association is causal. For example, the cessation of cigarette smoking is associated with a reduction in the risk of lung cancer relative to that in people who continue to smoke (see Figure 8.5). This finding strengthens the likelihood that cigarette smoking causes lung cancer. If the cause leads to rapid irreversible changes that subsequently produce disease whether or not there is continued exposure, then reversibility cannot be a condition for causality.

Study design

The ability of a study design to prove causation is an important consideration. Table 5.3 outlines the different types of study and relative strengths in establishing causality. These study designs were introduced in Chapter 3; their use in providing evidence for causal relationships is discussed below.

Experimental studies

The best evidence comes from well-designed randomized controlled trials. However, evidence is rarely available from this type of study, and often only relates to the effects of treatment and prevention campaigns. Other experimental studies, such as field and community trials, are seldom used to study causation. Evidence comes most often from observational studies; almost all the evidence on the health consequences of smoking comes from observational studies.

Table 5.3. Relative ability of different types of study to "prove" causation

Type of study	Ability to "prove" causation
Randomized controlled trials	Strong
Cohort studies	Moderate
Case-control studies	Moderate
Cross-sectional studies	Weak
Ecological studies	Weak

Cohort studies

Cohort studies are the next best design because, when well conducted, bias is minimized. Again, they are not always available. Although case-control studies are subject to several forms of bias, the results from large, well-designed investigations of this kind provide good evidence for the causal nature of an association; judgements often have to be made in the absence of data from other sources.

Cross-sectional studies

Cross-sectional studies are less able to prove causation as they provide no direct evidence on the time sequence of events. However, the time sequence can often be inferred from the way exposure and effect data is collected. For instance, if it is clear that the health effect is recent and the exposure to the potential causes is recorded in a questionnaire, questions about the past may clearly identify exposures before the effect occurred.

Ecological studies

Ecological studies provide the weakest evidence for causality because of the danger of incorrect extrapolation to individuals from regional or national data. However, for certain exposures that cannot normally be measured individually (such as air pollution, pesticide residues in food, fluoride in drinking water), evidence from ecological studies is very important. When causal relationships have already been established, well-designed ecological studies can be very useful.[27]

However, there are rare occasions when ecological studies provide good evidence for establishing causation. One such example relates to epidemics of asthma deaths. In 1968 the sale of inhaled bronchodilators without prescription in England and Wales was stopped because the increase in asthma deaths in the period 1959–66 had been shown to coincide with a rise in bronchodilator sales. After the availability of inhaled bronchodilators was restricted, the death rate fell. A similar pattern was observed following restrictions on the availability of the inhaled bronchodilator fenoterol in New Zealand in 1989.[28]

Judging the evidence

Regrettably, there are no completely reliable criteria for determining whether an association is causal or not. Causal inference is usually tentative and judgements must be made on the basis of the available evidence: uncertainty always remains. Evidence is often conflicting and due weight must be given to the different types when decisions are made. In judging the different aspects of causation referred to above, the correct temporal relationship is essential; once that has been established, the greatest weight may be given to plausibility, consistency and the dose–response relationship. The likelihood of a causal association is heightened when many different types of evidence lead to the same conclusion.

Evidence from well-designed studies is particularly important, especially if they are conducted in a variety of locations. The most important use of information about causation of diseases and injuries may be in the area of prevention, which we will discuss in the following chapters. When the causal pathways are established on the basis of quantitative information from epidemiological studies, the decisions about prevention may be uncontroversial. In situations where the causation is not so well established, but the impacts have great potential public health importance, the "precautionary principle"[29] may be applied to take preventive action as a safety measure; this is called "precautionary prevention".

Study questions

5.1 What is causal inference?

5.2 What is meant by a "hierarchy of causes"? List the components of this hierarchy for a specific disease.

5.3 Use the data in Table 1.2 to calculate the attributable fractions of smoking and asbestos exposure for lung cancer. If these fractions are added, the result is higher than 100%. Explain why this is important for the assessment of prevention approaches. What additional data is needed to calculate the population-attributable risk for each of the two exposures?

5.4 List the considerations commonly used to assess the causal nature of observed associations.

5.5 A statistically significant association has been demonstrated in a case-control study between the use of a drug for asthma and young people's risk of dying from asthma. What more do you need to know before you recommend the withdrawal of the drug?

5.6 During an outbreak of severe neurological disease of unknown cause, the families of the patients suggest that the cause is adulterated cooking oil of a particular brand. Based on considerations for causality in Table 5.1, what would you try to demonstrate first? What type of study would be suitable? At what stage would you intervene if the accumulating evidence showed that the oil might be the cause?

5.7 Why is time-series analysis of short-term associations between an environmental exposure (such as hot weather) and mortality considered an acceptable method to assess causality?

5.8 What is meant by meta-analysis, and which conditions have to be met for this to be applied to a set of studies?

5.9 By combining the data in Figure 5.8 and Figure 5.9, you can calculate a dose-relationship for income level and ischaemic heart disease (IHD) mediated by fruit and vegetable consumption (FVC). Assuming that the upper and lower quintiles in Figure 5.8 for FVC correspond to the upper and lower two deciles in Figure 5.9, what would be the combined relative risk for IHD in the highest versus the lowest quintile of FVC in a population? Suggest public health actions that can reduce additional risk for the low-income groups.

References

1. Rothman KJ, Greenland S. Causation and causal inference in epidemiology. *Am J Public Health* 2005;95:S144-50.

2. Marmot MG. The importance of psychosocial factors in the workplace to the development of disease. In: Marmot MG, Wilkinson RG, eds. *Social determinants of health*. New York, Oxford University Press, 1999.

3. Marmot M. Social determinants of health inequalities. *Lancet* 2005;365:1099-104.

4. Hosseinpoor AR, Mohammad K, Majdzadeh R, Naghavi M, Abolhassani F, Sousa A, et al. Socioeconomic inequality in infant mortality in Iran and across its provinces. *Bull World Health Organ* 2005;83:837-44.

5. Armstrong T, Bonita R. Capacity building for an integrated noncommunicable disease risk factor surveillance system in developing countries. *Ethn Dis* 2003;13:S13-8.

6. Kjellstrom T, van Kerkhoff L, Bammer G, McMichael T. Comparative assessment of transport risks — how it can contribute to health impact assessment of transport policies. *Bull World Health Organ* 2003;81:451-7.

7. *Introduction and methods - Assessing the environmental burden of disease at national and local levels*. Geneva, World Health Organization, 2003. (http://www.who.int/quantifying_ehimpacts/publications/en/.

8. Briggs D. *Making a difference: Indicators to improve children's environmental health*. Geneva, World Health Organization, 2003.

9. Weed DL. Causal criteria and Popperian refutation. In: Rothman JK, ed. *Causal Inference*. Massachusetts, Epidemiology Resources Inc, 1988.

10. *Smoking and health: report of the advisory committee to the Surgeon General of the Public Health Service* (PHS Publication No. 1103). Washington, United States Public Health Service,1964.

11. Hill AB. The environment and disease: association or causation? *Proc R Soc Med* 1965;58:295-300.

12. Mcmichael AJ, Campbell-Lendrum DH, Corvalan CF, Ebi KL, Githeko AK, Scheraga JD, et al. *Climate change and human health, risks and responses.* Geneva, World Health Organization, 2003.

13. Smith PG. The epidemics of bovine spongiform encephalopathy and variant Creutzfeldt-Jakob disease: current status and future prospects. *Bull World Health Organ* 2003;81:123-30.

14. Tong S, Baghurst P, McMichael A, Sawyer M, Mudge J. Low-level exposure to lead and children's intelligence at ages eleven to thirteen years: the Port Pirie cohort study. *BMJ* 1996;312:1569-75.

15. Meyer PA, Pivetz T, Dignam TA, Homa DM, Schoonover J, Brody D. Surveillance for elevated blood lead levels among children in the United States, 1997 – 2000. *MMWR* 2003;52:1-21.

16. Canfield RL, Henderson CR, Cory-Slechta DA, Cox C, Jusko TA, & Lanphear BP. Intellectual impairment in children with blood lead concentrations below 100 ug/l. *N Engl J Med* 2003;348:1517-26.

17. Wright NJ, Thacher TD, Pfitzner MA, Fischer PR, Pettifor JM. Causes of lead toxicity in a Nigerian city. *Arch Dis Child* 2005;90:262-6.

18. Sacks HS, Berrier J, Reitman D, Ancona-Berk VA, Chalmers TC. Meta-analysis of randomised controlled trials. *N Engl J Med* 1987;316:450-5.

19. Jadad AR, Cook DJ, Jones A, Klassen TP, Tugwell P, Moher M, et al. Methodology and reports of systematic reviews and meta–analyses: a comparison of Cochrane reviews with articles published in paper–based journals. *JAMA* 1998;280:278-80.

20. Little J, Cardy A, Munger RG. Tobacco smoking and oral clefts: a meta-analysis. *Bull World Health Organ* 2004;82:213-8.

21. Samet JM, Dominici F, Curriero FC, Coursac I, Zeger SL. Fine particle air pollution and mortality in 20 US cities. *N Engl J Med* 2000;343:1742-9.

22. Bell ML, Dominici F, Samet JM. A meta-analysis of time-series studies of ozone and mortality with comparison to the national morbidity, mortality and air pollution study. *Epidemiology* 2005;16:436-45.

23. Rose G. Sick individuals and sick populations. *Int J Epidemiol* 1985;14:32-8.

24. *The World Health Report: Reducing risks, Promoting Healthy Life.* Geneva, World Health Organization, 2002.

25. Department for food, environmental and rural affairs. *National food survey 2000.* London, The Stationery Office, 2001.

26. Robertson A, Tirado C, Lobstein T, Jermini M, Knai C, Jensen JH, et al., eds. *Food and health in Europe: a new basis for action.* WHO Regional Publications, European Series, No. 96. Copenhagen, World Health Organization, 2004.

27. Pearce NE. The ecologic fallacy strikes back. *J Epidemiol Community Health* 2000;54:326-7.

28. Pearce N, Hensley MJ. Beta agonists and asthma deaths. *Epidemiol Rev* 1998;20:173-86.

29. Grandjean P, Bailar J, Gee D, Needleman HL, Ozonoff DM, Richter E, et al. Implications of the precautionary principle in research and policy-making. *Am J Ind Med* 2004;45:382-5.

Chapter 6
Epidemiology and prevention: chronic noncommunicable diseases

Key messages

- Chronic noncommunicable diseases are major public health challenges in most countries.
- The causes of chronic diseases are generally known and cost-effective interventions are available.
- A comprehensive approach is required for the prevention and control of these diseases.
- Ultimately, primary prevention and control is the best strategy for the prevention of modern epidemics.
- Targeting high-risk individuals with secondary and tertiary prevention are also ways to reduce the burden of chronic disease.

The scope of prevention

The decline in death rates that occurred during the nineteenth century in high-income countries was principally due to a decrease in deaths from infectious disease.

Figure 6.1 shows tuberculosis death rates in England and Wales for the period 1840–1968 and indicates the times of introduction of specific preventive and therapeutic measures. Most of the decline in mortality took place before these interventions and has been attributed to improvements in nutrition, housing, sanitation and other environmental health measures.

Recent trends in death rates

In the last decades of the twentieth century, the declines in death rates from cardiovascular disease have accelerated in high-income countries. Since the 1970s, death rates from heart disease and stroke have fallen by up to 70% in Australia, Canada, Japan, the United Kingdom and the United States of America. There have also been improvements in cardiovascular mortality rates in middle-income countries, such as Poland. These gains have been the result of a wide range of measures directed at both whole populations and individuals. The preventive potential for chronic diseases is enormous. (Box 6.1). A decline in death rates of an additional 2% per annum over 10 years has the potential to avert the untimely deaths of 35 million people.[2]

[handwritten margin note: Important to know history of disease but as always improvements in things outside specific interventions can also have a great impact in prevalence of disease / ill health]

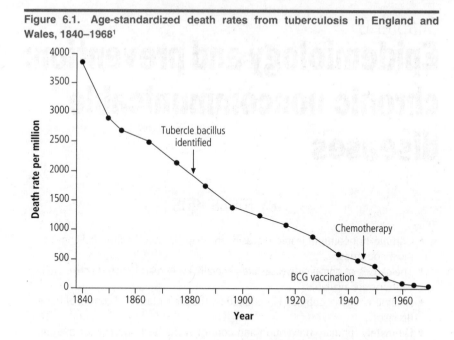

Figure 6.1. Age-standardized death rates from tuberculosis in England and Wales, 1840–1968[1]

The respective contributions of chronic and infectious conditions to total mortality has changed in the last century. For example, in Brazil infectious diseases accounted for 45% of all deaths in 1930, but only 5% in 2003 (Figure 6.2). In contrast, the proportion attributed to cardiovascular diseases increased from 12% in 1930 to 31% in 2003.

Figure 6.2. Changes in contribution of chronic and infectious conditions to total mortality in Brazilian state capitals, 1930–2005[8]

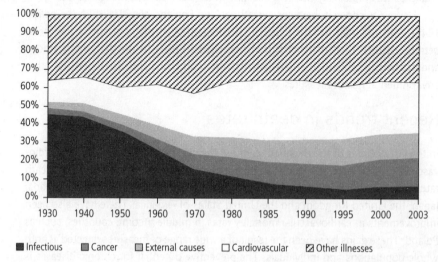

Proportional mortality in Brazilian state capitals

- Infectious diseases:
  46% in 1930
  5% in 2003

- Cardiovascular disease:
  12% in 1930
  31% in 2003

■ Infectious ■ Cancer ■ External causes □ Cardiovascular ▨ Other illnesses

However, mortality rates are influenced over time by the changing age structure of the population, as well as by waxing and waning epidemics. The changes in mortality rates in high-income countries have been particularly dramatic in the youngest age groups, where infectious diseases used to account for most mortality. Traffic accidents are now the leading cause of death in childhood in many high-income countries.

Preventive potential

The changing patterns of mortality and morbidity indicate that major causes of disease are preventable. Yet even the healthiest person will succumb at some age, and the lifetime mortality risk for any population is 100%. However, most populations are affected by specific diseases which can be prevented. Studies of migrants show that they often develop the patterns of disease of host populations. For example, the rates of gastric cancer in people born in Hawaii to Japanese parents are lower than those of people born in Japan. After two generations in the USA, people of Japanese heritage have the same gastric cancer rate as the US population in general. The fact that it takes a generation or more for the rates to fall suggests the importance of an exposure – such as diet – in early life.

[handwritten margin note: example of how studying environment can impact on type of intervention although some pop more susceptible there will usually be ↑ contributing factors]

Box 6.1. Chronic disease epidemiology: the basis of prevention

Chronic diseases are the major cause of death in almost all countries and account for 36 million deaths each year (see Figure 7.1). This translates to 61% of the world's deaths and 48% of the global burden of disease.[3] 20% of chronic noncommunicable disease deaths occur in high-income countries, and 80% occur in low- and middle-income countries – where most of the world's population live.

The leading chronic diseases are:

- cardiovascular disease (CVD), especially coronary heart disease and stroke (17.5 million deaths);
- cancer (7.5 million deaths);
- chronic respiratory disease (4 million deaths); and
- diabetes (1.1 million deaths).

Regional estimates indicate that chronic diseases are more frequent causes of death than communicable diseases worldwide, with the exception of the African region.

Injuries – accounting for almost one in ten deaths – feature prominently in all regions, caused mostly by traffic crashes, occupational injuries and interpersonal violence. The burden of injuries is increasing in most low- and middle-income countries.

Mental health problems are leading contributors to the burden of disease in many countries and contribute significantly to the incidence and severity of many chronic diseases, including cardiovascular diseases and cancer. Visual impairment and blindness, hearing impairment and deafness, oral diseases and genetic disorders are other chronic conditions that account for a substantial portion of the global burden of disease.

Without greater attention to prevention, it has been estimated that by 2030 myocardial infarct, stroke and diabetes will account for four in ten deaths among adults (35–64 years) in low- and middle-income countries, compared with one in eight deaths in the same age group in the United States of America and other high-income countries.[4] Projections suggest that over the next 10 years deaths due to chronic noncommunicable diseases will increase by 17%. This means that of the projected 64 million people who will die in 2015, 41 million will die of a chronic disease. However, large-scale prevention is feasible, as the causes of the major chronic diseases are known and are the same in all regions and population sub groups.[5-7] A small number of modifiable risk factors explain the most new cases, and evidence-based interventions are available, cost-effective and widely applicable.

Geographical variation in disease occurrence within and between countries also provides important clues to preventive potential (Figure 6.3). In the United Kingdom age-standardized male lung cancer rates fell from 18 per 100 000 in 1950 to 4 per 100 000 by 2000. In contrast, over the same period of time in France, male lung cancer rates increased. In France, the increase in tobacco use occurred some decades later than in the United Kingdom, and smoking rates started to decrease only after 1990. Similarly, global lung cancer rates in women continue to rise, but this increase has been avoided in the United Kingdom.[10]

Figure 6.3. Changes in lung cancer mortality at ages 35–44 in the United Kingdom and France, 1950–1999[9]

a) United Kingdom

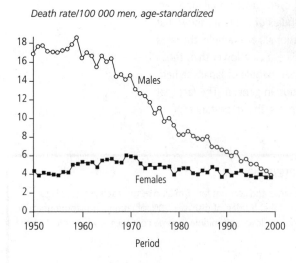

b) France

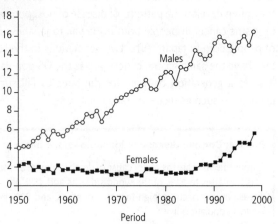

Causation framework

Epidemiology helps to identify modifiable causes of disease. Fifty years of epidemiological studies of coronary heart disease have identified much about the causes, from individual risk factors to cellular mechanisms in the arterial wall. However, the large differences between populations in risk factor levels are still not well understood. Causal inference needs to account both for disease-causation in the individual and for the social, economic, environmental and political contributions – the so-called upstream determinants – that are beyond the control of individuals (Figure 6.4).

Social determinants of health

The social determinants of health are the conditions in which people live and work.[14] Addressing the social determinants of health is the fairest way to improve health

> **Box 6.2. Effect of risk factor burden on lifetime risk**
>
> Epidemiologists investigate how the presence (or absence) of major risk factors contribute to the decline in death rates from cardiovascular diseases.[11,12] The absence of established risk factors at age 50 is associated with a very low lifetime risk of cardiovascular diseases. For example, an analysis of Framingham participants who were free of cardiovascular diseases at age 50 showed that the presence of 2 or more major risk factors conferred a lifetime risk of eventually developing cardiovascular disease of 69% in men and 50% in women. In comparison, those participants who had optimal risk profiles had lifetime risks of only 5.2% (men) and 8.2% (women) of developing cardiovascular disease.[13]

for all people. Good medical care is vital, but the factors that can undermine people's health – such as social position, housing conditions and occupational risks – need to be addressed to achieve equitable well being[15,16] Unfavourable social and environmental conditions may also lead to adverse behaviours, which can effect the levels of major risk factors for the main chronic diseases (Figure 6.4).

health for all
vs interventions
for targeted
groups

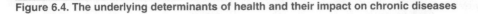

Figure 6.4. The underlying determinants of health and their impact on chronic diseases

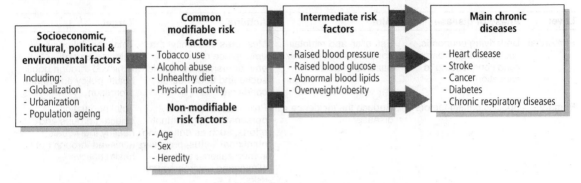

Public health nurses, medical sociologists, psychologists, health economists, ergonometrists, sanitary engineers, pollution control experts and occupational hygienists are all involved in disease-prevention efforts. As the limits of curative medicine become apparent and the costs of medical care escalate in all countries, disease prevention is gaining prominence.

Levels of prevention

The four levels of prevention, corresponding to different phases in the development of disease, are primordial, primary, secondary and tertiary.

Each of these levels targets factors or conditions which have an established role in causing disease. In situations where the evidence of such a role is incomplete, but the risk of not preventing a public health threat is deemed too high, preventive actions may still be taken and can be labelled "precautionary prevention." This approach is common in the environmental field, where the "precautionary principle" is used to avoid public health risks from processes or products.[17]

Approaches to prevention overlap and merge, yet all levels are important and complementary. Primordial and primary prevention contribute most to the health of the whole population, while secondary and tertiary prevention are generally focused on people who already have signs of disease (Table 6.1).

Primordial prevention

This level of prevention was identified as a result of increasing knowledge about the epidemiology of cardiovascular diseases. It is known that coronary heart disease occurs on a large scale only if the basic underlying cause is present, i.e. a diet high in saturated animal fat. Where this cause is largely absent – as in China and Japan – coronary heart disease remains a rare cause of mortality and morbidity, despite the high frequencies of other important risk factors such as cigarette smoking and high blood pressure. However, smoking-induced lung cancer is on the increase and strokes induced by high blood pressure are common in China and Japan. In some middle-income countries, cardiovascular disease is becoming important in the urban middle- and upper-income groups, who have already acquired high-risk behaviour. As socioeconomic development occurs, such risk factors can be expected to become

Table 6.1. Levels of prevention

Level	Phase of disease	Aim	Actions	Target
Primordial	Underlying economic, social, and environmental conditions leading to causation	Establish and maintain conditions that minimize hazards to health	Measures that inhibit the emergence of environmental, economic, social and behavioural conditions.	Total population or selected groups; achieved through public health policy and health promotion.
Primary	Specific causal factors	Reduce the incidence of disease	Protection of health by personal and communal efforts, such as enhancing nutritional status, providing immunizations, and eliminating environmental risks.	Total population, selected groups and healthy individuals; achieved through public health policy.
Secondary	Early stage of disease	Reduce the prevalence of disease by shortening its duration	Measures available to individuals and communities for early detection and prompt intervention to control disease and minimize disability (e.g. through screening programs).	Individuals at high risk and patients; achieved through preventive medicine.
Tertiary	Late stage of disease (treatment, rehabilitation)	Reduce the number and/or impact of complications	Measures aimed at softening the impact of long-term disease and disability; minimizing suffering; maximizing potential years of useful life.	Patients; achieved through rehabilitation.

more widespread. The aim of primordial prevention (Box 6.3) is to avoid the emergence and establishment of the social, economic and cultural patterns of living that are known to contribute to an elevated risk of disease.

The importance of primordial prevention is often realized too late. All countries need to avoid the spread of unhealthy lifestyles and consumption patterns. Primordial prevention of chronic disease should include national policies and programmes on nutrition. Such programmes need to involve the agricultural sector, the food industry and the food import/export sector. Countries also need programmes to promote regular physical activity. The example of tobacco use indicates that a high level of government commitment is required for effective primordial prevention. There is good evidence that tobacco consumption can be reduced by taxation and increased prices (Figure 6.5). The epidemiological evidence showing the harmful effects of tobacco use ultimately led to the Framework Convention on Tobacco Control in February 2006, the first health treaty adopted by the Member States of the World Health Organization (see Chapter 10).

Box 6.3. Preventing air pollution

Primordial prevention is needed to counter the global effects of air pollution, such as the greenhouse effect, acid rain, ozone-layer depletion and the health effects of smog. Atmospheric particulate matter and sulfur dioxide concentrations in many major cities exceed the maximum recommended by the World Health Organization and the United Nations Environment Programme (UNEP). Cities in low- and middle-income countries that rely on coal as an energy supply are particularly affected. Public policies aimed at preventing these hazards are needed in most countries to protect health (see Chapter 9). Primordial prevention includes city planning that separates industrial from residential areas, facilitates public or "active" transport (walking, bicycling) and encourages energy conservation.

Figure 6.5. Inverse relation between real price of cigarettes and cigarette consumption, South Africa, 1961–2001[3]

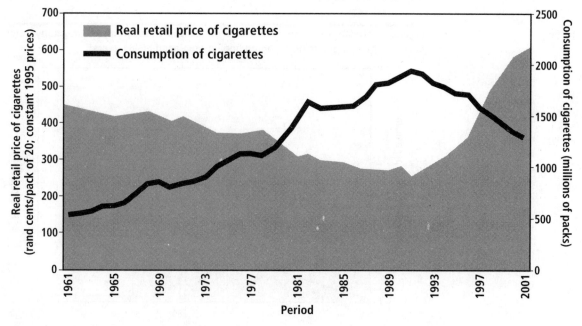

Primary prevention

The purpose of primary prevention is to limit the incidence of disease by controlling specific causes and risk factors. Primary prevention efforts can be directed at:

- the whole population with the aim of reducing average risk (the population or "mass" strategy); or
- people at high risk as a result of particular exposures (the high-risk-individual strategy).

Population strategy

The population approach aims to shift the whole population distribution to the left on an imaginary x-axis; i.e. to reduce the mean population level of cholesterol (or blood pressure). The major advantage of the population strategy is that one does not have to identify the high-risk group but simply aim to reduce – by a small amount – the level of a given risk factor in the entire population. Its main disadvantage is that it offers little benefit to many individuals because their absolute risks of disease are quite low. For example, most people will wear a seat-belt while driving a car for their entire life without being involved in a crash. The widespread wearing of seat-belts has been very beneficial to the population as a whole, but little apparent benefit is accrued by those individuals who are never personally involved in a crash. This phenomenon has been called the prevention paradox.[18]

The high incidence of cardiovascular disease in most industrialized countries is due to the high levels of risk factors in the population as a whole, not to the problems of a minority. The relationship between serum cholesterol and the risk of coronary heart disease (Figure 6.6), shows that the distribution of cholesterol is skewed a little

Figure 6.6. Relationship between serum cholesterol (histogram) and mortality from coronary heart disease (interrupted line) in men aged 55–64 years[19]

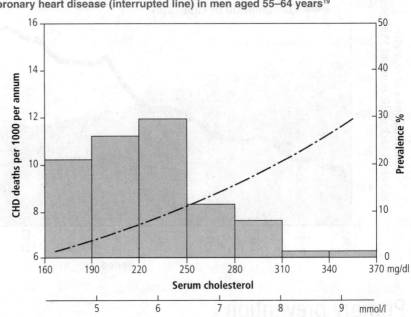

to the right. Only a small minority of the population have a serum cholesterol level above 8 mmol/l, i.e. a very high risk of coronary heart disease. Most of the deaths attributable to coronary heart disease occur in the middle range of the cholesterol level, where most of the population is. In this case, primary prevention depends on changes that reduce the average risk in the whole population, thus shifting the whole distribution to a lower level.

Figure 6.7 compares the distribution of total cholesterol in three populations with different means. There is little overlap between people with high cholesterol levels in population A and population C. People with high cholesterol in population A would be considered to have low levels in population C.

These data come from the WHO MONICA (MONItoring of trends and determinants in CArdiovascular disease) Project, which comprised population surveys done at least twice in a decade in 38 geographically defined populations in 21 countries.[12, 20]

The figure also illustrates the principle that any cut-off point for determining prevalence is arbitrary, but shifting the population mean by a small amount has a large impact. Shifting the population distribution from high levels to low levels is the purpose of primary prevention. In Figure 6.7, we can observe that:

- Population A with low mean cholesterol (4.0 mmol/l) also has a low prevalence of hypercholesterolaemia (6%), even if the cut-off point for determining prevalence is set at ≥ 5.0 mmol/l.

- Population B with a mean cholesterol of 5.4 mmol/l would classify almost two thirds of the population (64%) as having "high" cholesterol if the cut-off point were ≥ 5.0 mmol/l, but only 15% if the cut-off point were 6.2 mmol/l.
- The area under the curve in population C includes almost everyone if the cut-off point is set as low as ≥ 5.0 mmol/l.

Figure 6.7. Total cholesterol (mmol/l) distribution in three populations: A (low), B (average) and C (high).[21]

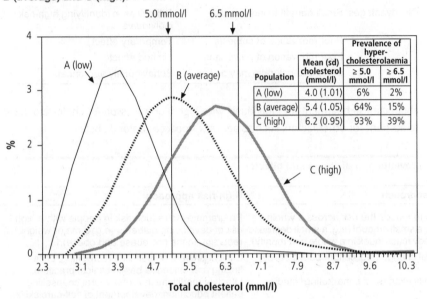

Population	Mean (sd) cholesterol (mmol/l)	Prevalence of hyper-cholesterolaemia	
		≥ 5.0 mmol/l	≥ 6.5 mmol/l
A (low)	4.0 (1.01)	6%	2%
B (average)	5.4 (1.05)	64%	15%
C (high)	6.2 (0.95)	93%	39%

High-risk individual strategy

The alternative approach is to focus on individuals above an arbitrary cut-off point in an attempt to reduce the cholesterol levels in those individuals. Although the high-risk-individual strategy (which aims to protect susceptible persons) is most efficient for the people at greatest risk of a specific disease, these people may contribute little to the overall burden of the disease in the population. However, if people with established disease are included in this high-risk group, the strategy will contribute more to the overall reduction in the burden of disease (Box 6.4). The main disadvantage of the high-risk-individual strategy is that it usually requires a screening programme to identify the high-risk group, something that is often difficult and costly. Table 6.2 lists the advantages and disadvantages of the two strategies.

Combining the population strategy and a high-risk strategy is useful in many situations. Table 6.3 compares both approaches to the prevention of diabetes and obesity. The high-risk strategy is also more relevant when focused on individuals at high overall risk rather than those at high risk in terms of a single risk factor. For example, decisions

> **Box 6.4. High-risk strategy: smoking cessation**
>
> Smoking cessation programmes provide an excellent example of a high-risk strategy and are appropriate since most smokers wish to abandon the habit; thus individual smokers and the physicians concerned are usually strongly motivated. The benefits of intervention directed at high-risk individuals are likely to outweigh any adverse effects, such as the short-term effects of nicotine withdrawal. If the high-risk strategy is successful, it also benefits nonsmokers by reducing their passive smoking. Such programmes are more likely to be effective when complemented by population approaches to tobacco control.

Table 6.2. Advantages and disadvantages of primary prevention strategies[18, 22]

Feature	Population strategy	High-risk-individual strategy
Advantages	Radical	Appropriate for individuals
	Large potential for whole population	Subject motivation
	Behaviourally appropriate	Physician motivation
		Favourable benefit-to-risk ratio
Disadvantages	Small benefit to individuals	Difficulties in identifying high-risk individuals
	Poor motivation of subjects	Temporary effect
	Poor motivation of physicians	Limited effect
	Benefit-to-risk ratio may be low	Behaviourally appropriate

about clinical treatment for individuals with high blood pressure or cholesterol need to account for other factors such as age, sex, tobacco use or diabetes.

Table 6.3. Approaches to the prevention of diabetes and obesity

Feature	Population approach	High-risk approach
Description	Programmes to reduce the risk across a whole population by a small amount (e.g. a small decrease in average body mass index in a whole community).	Programmes to reduce risk in people with a high risk of developing diabetes (e.g. a major weight reduction in the pre-obese and obese).
Techniques	Environmental change (legislation, public policy, pricing); Lifestyle modification (social marketing, media advocacy).	Clinical prevention services (screening, case-finding and evidence-based clinical practice); Lifestyle modification (behavioural counselling, patient education, development of self-care skills).
Impact	Improved behavioural patterns across the whole population, caused partly by automatic choices due to supportive environments (pedestrian-only areas increase physical activity by default among people who frequent those areas).	Reduced disease incidence among people at high risk (reduced stroke among people treated for hypertension, or reduced diabetes among people with impaired glucose tolerance due to intensive lifestyle change).
Cost	Small cost per person multiplied by large population.	High cost per person for a relatively small number of persons.
Timing of results	Impact on lifestyle is seen in the short-term (reduced fat intake follows automatically after a food product's composition is reformulated; tobacco consumption falls immediately after effective legislative measures are enforced).	Impact on lifestyle seen within one to two years of initiating programme of intensive education, counselling, support and follow-up. Medium-term outcomes of reduced disease incidence seen for diabetes.

Secondary prevention

Secondary prevention aims to reduce the more serious consequences of disease through early diagnosis and treatment. It comprises the measures available to individuals and populations for early detection and effective intervention. It is directed at the period between the onset of disease and the normal time of diagnosis, and aims to reduce the prevalence of disease.

Secondary prevention can be applied only to diseases in which the natural history includes an early period when it is easily identified and treated, so that progression to a more serious stage can be stopped. The two main requirements for a useful secondary prevention programme are a safe and accurate method of detecting the disease – preferably at a preclinical stage – and effective methods of intervention.

Cervical cancer provides an example of the importance of secondary prevention and of the difficulties of assessing the value of prevention programmes.

Figure 6.8 shows an association between screening rates and reductions in the death rate from cervical cancer in selected Canadian provinces in the 1970s.[23, 24] The data were initially questioned because the mortality rates for cervical cancer were already decreasing before organized screening programmes started. Other studies have since supported the value of such screening programmes, which are now widely applied in many – but not all – countries. Few low- and middle-income countries have the infrastructure for organized screening programs, and most women in low-income countries do not have access to routine screening.[25] With the advent of an effective vaccine for human papillomavirus, cervical cancer is likely to become an example of a disease for which primary prevention measures predominate.

Figure 6.8. Relationship between decrease in death rates from cancer of the cervix between 1960–62 and 1970–72 and population screening rates in Canadian provinces[23, 24]

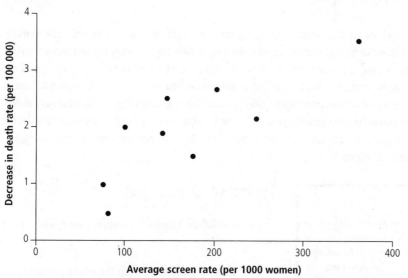

Other examples of secondary prevention measures that are widely used include testing of eyesight and hearing in school-age children, screening for high blood pressure in middle age, testing for hearing loss in factory workers, and skin testing and chest radiographs for the diagnosis of tuberculosis.

Tertiary prevention

Tertiary prevention is aimed at reducing the progress or complications of established disease and is an important aspect of therapeutic and rehabilitation medicine. It consists of the measures intended to reduce impairments and disabilities, minimize suffering caused by poor health and promote patients' adjustment to incurable conditions. Tertiary prevention is often difficult to separate from treatment, since the treatment of chronic disease has as one of its central aims the prevention of recurrence.

The rehabilitation of patients with poliomyelitis, strokes, injuries, blindness and other chronic conditions is essential to their ability to take part in daily social life. Tertiary prevention can improve individual and family well being and income. An important aspect of tertiary prevention – particularly for younger people afflicted by illness or injury – is restoring their ability to work and earn a livelihood. If welfare systems are not functioning, even a temporary period of ill-health may cause severe economic hardship for the patient and his or her family. Epidemiological studies need to include the economic situation of people with ill-health as one of the crucial social determinants of health outcomes.

Screening

Screening people for disease – or risk factors which predict disease – is motivated by the potential benefits of secondary prevention through early detection and treatment.

Definition

Screening is the process of using tests on a large scale to identify the presence of disease in apparently healthy people. Screening tests do not usually establish a diagnosis, but rather the presence or absence of an identified risk factor, and thus require individual follow-up and treatment. As the recipients of screening are usually people who have no illness it is important that the screening test itself is very unlikely to cause harm.[26] Screening can also be used to identify high exposure to risk factors. For instance, children's blood samples can be screened for lead in areas of high use of lead in paint.

Types of screening

There are different types of screening, each with specific aims:

- *mass screening* aims to screen the whole population (or subset);
- *multiple* or *multiphasic screening* uses several screening tests at the same time;
- *targeted screening* of groups with specific exposures, e.g. workers in lead battery factories, is often used in environmental and occupational health (Box 6.5); and
- *case-finding* or *opportunistic screening* is aimed at patients who consult a health practitioner for some other purpose.

Box 6.5. Targeted screening

When targeted screening is done in groups with occupational exposures, the criteria for screening are not necessarily as strict as those for general population screening. The health effect that is prevented may be minor (nausea or headache), but screening may be a high priority if the effect reduces the patient's ability to work. Many health effects from exposure to environmental hazards are graded, and preventing a minor effect may also prevent more serious effects. Targeted screening can be legally required – for example, in miners or people working with lead or chromium – and used in the follow-up to environmental pollution incidents, such as methyl-mercury poisoning (Minamata disease) in Japan in the 1960s (see Chapter 1 and Chapter 9).

Criteria for screening

Table 6.4 lists the main criteria for establishing a screening programme.[27] These relate to the characteristics of the disorder or disease, its treatment and the screening test.

Above all, the disease should be one that would prove serious if not diagnosed early; inborn metabolic defects such as phenylketonuria meet this criterion, as do some cancers, such as cancer of the cervix.

Table 6.4. Requirements for instituting a medical screening programme

Disorder	Well-defined
Prevalence	Known
Natural history	Long period between first signs and overt disease; medically important disorder for which there is an effective remedy
Test choice	Simple and safe
Test performance	Distributions of test values in affected and unaffected individuals known
Financial	Cost-effective
Facilities	Available or easily provided
Acceptability	Procedures following a positive result are generally agreed upon and acceptable to both the screening authorities and to those screened.
Equity	Equity of access to screening services; effective, acceptable and safe treatment available

---

In addition, several issues need to be addressed before establishing a screening programme.

Costs

The costs of a screening programme must be balanced against the number of cases detected and the consequences of not screening. Generally, the prevalence of the preclinical stage of the disease should be high in the population screened, but occasionally it may be worthwhile to screen even for diseases of low prevalence which have serious consequences, such as phenylketonuria. If children with phenylketonuria are identified at birth, they can be given a special diet that will allow them to develop normally. If they are not given the diet, they become mentally retarded and require special care throughout life. In spite of the low incidence of this metabolic disease (2–4 per 100 000 births), secondary prevention screening programmes are highly cost-effective.

Lead time

The disease must have a reasonably long lead time; that is, the interval between the time when the disease can be first diagnosed by screening and when it is usually diagnosed in patients presenting with symptoms. Noise-induced hearing loss has a very long lead time; pancreatic cancer usually has a short one. A short lead time implies a rapidly progressing disease, and treatment initiated after screening is unlikely to be more effective than that begun after the more usual diagnostic procedures.

Length bias

Early treatment should be more effective in reducing mortality or morbidity than treatment begun after the development of overt disease, as, for example, in the treatment of cervical cancer in situ. A treatment must be effective and acceptable to people who are asymptomatic. If treatment is ineffective, earlier diagnosis only increases the time period during which the participant is aware of the disease; this effect is known as length bias or length/time bias.

Screening test

The screening test itself must be cheap, easy to apply, acceptable to the public, reliable and valid. A test is reliable if it provides consistent results, and valid if it correctly categorizes people into groups with and without disease, as measured by its sensitivity and specificity.

- *Sensitivity* is the proportion of people with the disease in the screened population who are identified as ill by the screening test. (When the disease is present, how often does the test detect it?)
- *Specificity* is the proportion of disease-free people who are so identified by the screening test. (When the disease is absent, how often does the test provide a negative result?)

The methods for calculating these measures and the positive and negative predictive values are given in Table 6.5.

Although a screening test ideally is both highly sensitive and highly specific, we need to strike a balance between these characteristics, because most tests cannot do both. We determine this balance by an arbitrary cut-off point between normal and abnormal. If we want to increase sensitivity and to include all true positives, we are obliged to increase the number of false positives, which means decreasing specificity. Reducing the strictness of the criteria for a positive test can increase sensitivity, but by doing this the test's specificity is reduced. Likewise, increasing the strictness of the criteria increases specificity but decreases sensitivity. We also need to account for predictive value when interpreting the results of screening tests.

Table 6.5. Validity of a screening test

		Disease status		
		Present	Absent	Total
Screening test	**Positive**	*a*	*b*	*a+b*
	Negative	*c*	*d*	*c+d*
	Total	*a+c*	*b+d*	*a+b+c+d*

a = No. of true positives, b = No. of false positives,
c = No. of false negatives, d = No. of true negatives

Sensitivity	= probability of a positive test in people with the disease = $a/(a+c)$
Specificity	= probability of a negative test in people without the disease = $d/(b+d)$
Positive predictive value	= probability of the person having the disease when the test is positive = $a/(a+b)$
Negative predictive value	= probability of the person not having the disease when the test is negative = $d/(c+d)$

Decisions on the appropriate criteria for a screening test depend on the consequences of identifying false negatives and false positives. For a serious condition in newborn children, it might be preferable to have high sensitivity and to accept the increased cost of a high number of false positives (reduced specificity). Further follow-up would then be required to identify the true positives and true negatives.

Natural history

Above all, establishing appropriate criteria requires considerable knowledge of the natural history of the disease in question and of the benefits and costs of treatment. Adequate facilities must exist for formal diagnosis, treatment and follow-up of newly diagnosed cases, which could otherwise overwhelm the health services. Finally, the screening policy and programme must be accepted by all the people involved: administrators, health professionals and the public.

Impact

The value of a screening programme is ultimately determined by its effect on morbidity, mortality and disability. Ideally, information should be available on disease rates in people whose disease was identified through screening and in those whose disease was diagnosed on the basis of symptoms. Because differences are likely to exist between people who take part in screening programmes and people who do not, the best evidence for the effectiveness of screening comes from the results of randomized controlled trials (Box 6.6).

> **Box 6.6. Breast cancer screening: a case study**
>
> A randomized controlled trial of 60 000 insured women aged 40–64 who were followed for up to 23 years found that mammography was effective in reducing mortality from breast cancer (Table 6.6). Ten years after entry into the study, the breast cancer mortality was about 29% lower among women who been screened than among those who had not; at 18 years, the rate was about 23% lower.

Table 6.6. Breast cancer mortality rates at follow-up[28]

	No. of women with breast cancer	No. of deaths (from start of follow-up)		
		5 years	10 years	18 years
Screened group	307	39	95	126
Control group	310	63	133	163
% difference		38.1	28.6	22.7

This *relative* reduction in mortality from breast cancer of 23%–29% looks less impressive when considered in *absolute* terms (the absolute mortality reduction was 0.05% of women screened). Another randomized control trial from the Swedish National Health Board showed a relative benefit of similar magnitude (31%), but also indicated that this represented a net benefit of 4 deaths averted for 10 000 women screened.

In these studies, the marginal improvement in terms of reduced mortality was only perceptible in women over 50 years of age. A much greater benefit in life-years gained would be achieved if screening mammography delayed death from breast cancer in younger women, but unfortunately this is not the case.[29]

Finally, the best preventive strategy does not necessarily include screening.[30] Where an important risk factor (such as tobacco use, raised blood pressure or physical inactivity) can be reduced without selecting a high-risk group for preventive action, it is better to concentrate on available resources and use public policy and environmental measures to establish mass approaches to prevention.

Study questions

6.1 Describe the four levels of prevention. Give examples of action at each level which would be appropriate as part of a comprehensive programme to prevent stroke.

6.2 Which of the two approaches to primary prevention of diabetes and obesity outlined in Table 6.3 is preferable?

6.3 What characteristics of a disease would indicate its suitability for screening?

6.4 What epidemiological study designs can be used to evaluate a screening programme?

References

1. Mckeown T. *The role of medicine: dream, mirage or nemesis?* London, Nuffield Provincial Hospitals Trust, 1976.

2. Strong K, Mathers C, Leeder S, Beaglehole R. Preventing chronic diseases: how many lives can we save? *Lancet* 2005;366:1578-82.

3. *Prevention of chronic diseases: a vital investment.* Geneva, World Health Organization, 2005.

4. Leeder SR, Raymond S. *Race against time.* New York, Columbia University, 2004.

5. Lopez AD, Mathers CD, Ezzati M, Jamison DT, Murray CJL. Global and regional burden of disease and risk factors, 2001: systematic analysis of population health data. *Lancet* 2006;367:1747-57.

6. Yusuf S, Hawken S, Ounpuu S, Dans T, Avezum A, Lanas F, et al. Effect of potentially modifiable risk factors associated with myocardial infarction in 52 countries (the INTERHEART study). *Lancet* 2004;364:937-52.

7. *The world health report: reducing risks, promoting healthy life.* Geneva, World Health Organization, 2002.

8. Rouquairol MZ, Almeida Filho N, editors. *Epidemiologia e Saúde.* Rio de Janeiro, Editora Medís, 1999.

9. Jamison DT, Breman JG, Measham AR, Alleyne G, Claeson M, Evans DB, et al. *Disease control priorities in developing countries,* 2nd ed. New York, Oxford University Press, 2006.

10. Peto R, Lopez AD, Boreham J, Thun J. *Mortality from smoking in developed countries,* 2nd ed. Oxford, Oxford University Press, 2003.

11. Critchley J, Liu J, Zhao D, Wei W, Capewell S. Explaining the increase in coronary heart disease mortality in Beijing between 1984 and 1999. *Circulation* 2004;110:1236-44.

12. Tunstall-Pedoe H, Vanuzzo D, Hobbs M, Mahonen M, Cepaitis Z, Kuulasmaa K, et al. Estimation of contribution of changes in coronary care to improving survival, event rates, and coronary heart disease mortality across the WHO MONICA Project populations. *Lancet* 2000;355:688-700.

13. Lloyd-Jones DM, Leip EP, Larson MG, D'Agostino RB, Beiser A, Wilson PW. Prediction of lifetime risk for cardiovascular disease by risk factor burden at 50 years of age. *Circulation* 2006;113:791-8.

14. Marmot M. Social determinants of health inequalities. *Lancet* 2005;365:1099-104.

15. Lee JW. Public health is a social issue. *Lancet* 2005;365:1685-6.

16. Bonita R, Irwin A, Beaglehole R. Promoting public health in the twenty-first century: the role of the World Health Organization. In: Kawachi I, Wamala S. eds. *Globalization and health*. Oxford, Oxford University Press, 2006.

17. Martuzzi M, Tickner JA. *The precautionary principle: protecting public health, the environment and the future of our children*. Copenhagen, World Health Organization Regional Office for Europe, 2004.

18. Rose G. Sick individuals and sick populations. *Int J Epidemiol* 1985;14:32-8.

19. Prevention of coronary heart disease: report of a WHO Expert Committee. *WHO Tech Rep Ser* 1982;678.

20. Tolonen H, Dobson A, Kulathinal S, Sangita A, for the WHO MONICA Project. Assessing the quality of risk factor survey data: lessons from the WHO MONICA Project. *Eur J Cardiovasc Prev Rehabil* 2006;13:104-14.

21. Tolonen H. *Towards high quality of population health surveys. Standardization and quality control*. Helsinki, National Public Health Institute, 2005. (http://www.ktl.fi/portal/4043)

22. Rose GA. *The strategy of preventive medicine*. Oxford, Oxford University Press, 1992.

23. Boyes DA, Nichols TM, Millner AM, Worth AJ. Recent results from the British Columbia screening program for cervical cancer. *Am J Obstet Gynecol* 1977;128:692-3.

24. Miller AB, Lindsay J, Hill GB. Mortality from cancer of the uterus in Canada and its relationship to screening for cancer of the cervix. *Int J Cancer* 1976;17:602-12.

25. Katz IT, Wright AA. Preventing cervical cancer in the developing world. *N Engl J Med* 2006;354:1110.

26. Wald NJ. Guidance on medical screening. *J Med Screen* 2001;8:56.

27. Cuckle HS, Wald NJ. Tests using single markers. In: Wald NI, Leck I, eds. *Antenatal and neonatal screening*. Oxford, Oxford University Press, 2000:20.

28. Shapiro S. Determining the efficacy of breast cancer screening. *Cancer* 1989;63:1873-80.

29. Wright C, Mueller C. Screening mammography and public health policy: the need for perspective. *Lancet* 1995;346:29-32.

30. Strong K, Wald N, Miller A, Alwan A. Current concepts in screening for non-communicable disease. *J Med Screen* 2005;12:12-9.

Chapter 7

Communicable diseases: epidemiology surveillance and response

Key messages

- New communicable diseases emerge and old ones re-emerge in the context of social and environmental change.
- Current burdens of communicable diseases make them a continuing threat to public health in all countries.
- Epidemiological methods enable surveillance, prevention and control of communicable disease outbreaks.
- The International Health Regulations aim to facilitate the control of new epidemics.

Introduction

Definitions

A communicable (or infectious) disease is one caused by transmission of a specific pathogenic agent to a susceptible host. Infectious agents may be transmitted to humans either:

- directly, from other infected humans or animals, or
- indirectly, through vectors, airborne particles or vehicles.

Vectors are insects or animals that carry the infectious agent from person to person. Vehicles are contaminated objects or elements of the environment (such as clothes, cutlery, water, milk, food, blood, plasma, parenteral solutions or surgical instruments).

Contagious diseases are those that can be spread (contagious literally means "by touch") between humans without an intervening vector or vehicle. Malaria is therefore a communicable but not a contagious disease, while measles and syphilis are both communicable and contagious. Some pathogens cause disease not only through infection but through the toxic effect of chemical compounds that these produce. For example, *Staphylococcus aureus* is a bacteria that can infect humans directly, but staphylococcal food poisoning is caused by ingestion of food contaminated with a toxin that the bacteria produces.

Role of epidemiology

Epidemiology developed from the study of outbreaks of communicable disease and of the interaction between agents, hosts, vectors and reservoirs. The ability to describe the circumstances that tend to spark epidemics in human populations – war, migration, famine and natural disasters – has increased human ability to control the spread of communicable disease through surveillance, prevention, quarantine and treatment.

The burden of communicable disease

The estimated global burden of communicable diseases – dominated by HIV/AIDS, tuberculosis and malaria – is shown in Box 7.1. Emerging diseases such as viral haemorrhagic fevers, new variant Creutzfeld-Jakob disease and severe acute respiratory syndrome (SARS), as well as re-emerging diseases including diphtheria, yellow fever, anthrax, plague, dengue and influenza place a large and unpredictable burden on health systems, particularly in low-income countries.

Threats to human security and health systems

Communicable diseases pose an acute threat to individual health and have the potential to threaten collective human security. While low-income countries continue to deal with the problems of communicable diseases, deaths due to chronic diseases are rapidly increasing, especially in urban settings (see Chapter 6). Although high-income countries have proportionally less communicable disease mortality, these countries still bear the costs of high morbidity from certain communicable diseases. For example, in high-income countries, upper respiratory tract infections cause significant mortality only at the extremes of age (in children and elderly people). However, the associated morbidity is substantial, and affects all age-groups (Figure 7.2).

Using epidemiological methods to investigate and control communicable disease is still a challenge for the health profession. Investigation must be done quickly and often with limited resources. The consequences of a successful investigation are rewarding, but failure to act

---

Box 7.1. Global burden of communicable disease

Communicable diseases account for 14.2 million deaths each year (Figure 7.1). Another 3.3 million deaths are attributable to maternal and perinatal conditions and nutritional deficiencies. Together these account for 30% of the world's deaths and 39% of the global burden of disability.[1]

Six causes account for almost half of all premature deaths, mostly in children and young adults, and account for almost 80% of all deaths from infectious diseases:

- Acute respiratory infections (3.76 million)
- HIV/AIDS (2.8 million)
- Diarrhoeal diseases (1.7 million)
- Tuberculosis (1.6 million)
- Malaria (1 million)
- Measles (0.8 million)

Most of these deaths occur in low-income countries. WHO projections suggest that – due to better prevention – total deaths from these causes will decline by 3% over the next 10 years.

Figure 7.1. Projected main causes of death worldwide, all ages, 2005: total deaths 58 million[1]

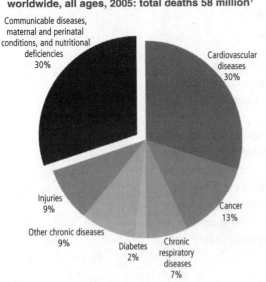

effectively can be damaging. In the AIDS pandemic, 25 years of pidemiological studies have helped to characterize the agent, modes of transmission and effective means of prevention. However, despite this knowledge, the estimated global prevalence of HIV in 2006 was 38.6 million cases, with 3 million deaths per year.

Epidemic and endemic disease

Epidemics

Epidemics are defined as the occurrence of cases in excess of what is normally expected in a community or region. When describing an epidemic, the time period, geographical region and particulars of the population in which the cases occur must be specified.

The number of cases needed to define an epidemic varies according to the agent, the size, type and suscep- tibility of population exposed, and the time and place of occurrence. The identification of an epidemic also de- pends on the usual frequency of the disease in the area among the specified population during the same season of the year. A very small number of cases of a disease not previously recognized in an area, but associated in time and place, may be sufficient to constitute an epidemic. For example, the first report on the syndrome that became known as AIDS concerned only four cases of *Pneumocys- tis carinii* pneumonia in young homosexual men.[3] Previ- ously this disease had been seen only in patients with compromised immune systems. The rapid development of the epidemic of Kaposi sarcoma, another manifestation of AIDS, in New York is shown in Figure 7.3: 2 cases occurred in 1977 and 1978 and by 1982 there were 88 cases.[3]

The dynamic of an epidemic is determined by the characteristics of its agent and its pattern of transmission, and by the susceptibility of its human hosts. The three main groups of pathogenic agents act very differently in this respect. A limited number of bacteria, viruses and parasites cause most epidemics, and a thorough understand- ing of their biology has improved specific prevention measures. Vaccines, the most effective means of preventing infectious diseases, have been developed so far only for some viral and bacterial diseases. If the attempt to make a malaria vaccine is successful, this will be the first vaccine for a parasitic disease. Vaccines work on both an individual basis, by preventing or attenuating clinical disease in a person exposed to the pathogen, and also on a population basis, by affecting herd immunity (Figure 7.4).

In a point-source epidemic, susceptible individuals are exposed more or less simultaneously to one source of infection. This results in a very rapid increase in the number of cases, often in a few hours. The cholera epidemic (a bacterial disease)

Figure 7.2. Projected main causes of burden of disease in disability adjusted life years (DALYs) by World Bank income group,[2] all ages, 2005

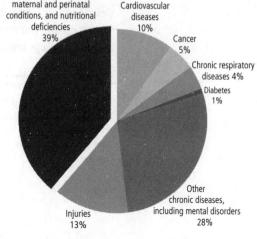

Figure 7.3. Kaposi sarcoma in New York[3]

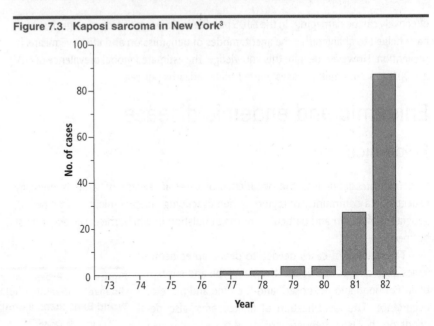

described in Chapter 1 is an example of a point-source epidemic, one in which effective control (by removing access to the source) was possible 30 years before the actual agent was identified (Figure 7.5).

Figure 7.4. Herd immunity. Black circles show individuals infected by a contagious disease, white circles are individuals who are not affected, and the grey circle represents the one person who was immune. The arrows show the direction of transmission. In A, all individuals were susceptible, and all were affected. In B, only one individual was immune, yet four were protected, even though three of them were susceptible.[5]

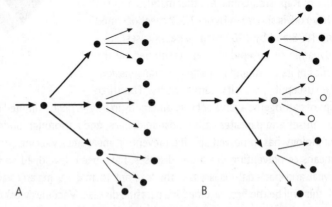

In a contagious, or propagated, epidemic the disease is passed from person to person and the initial rise in the number of cases is slower. The number of susceptible individuals and the potential sources of infection are the critical factors in determining the spread of disease. For example, SARS was first recognized as a global threat in March 2003. It spread rapidly to 26 countries, affecting adult men and women, with a fifth of all cases occurring among health-care workers (see Chapter 1).

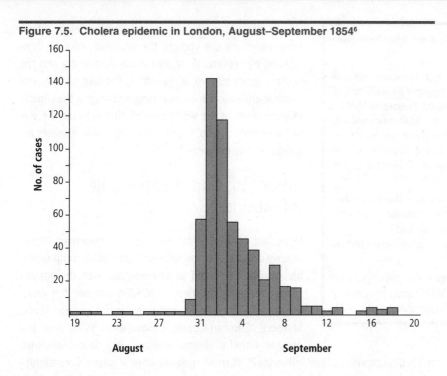

Figure 7.5. Cholera epidemic in London, August–September 1854[6]

Endemic diseases

Communicable diseases are termed endemic when they have a relatively stable pattern of occurrence in a given geographical area or population group at relatively high prevalence and incidence. Endemic diseases such as malaria are among the major health problems in low-income tropical countries. If conditions change in the host, the agent or the environment, an endemic disease may become epidemic. For example, improved smallpox control in Europe was reversed during the First World War (Table 7.1).

Table 7.1. Deaths from smallpox in selected European countries, 1900–1919

Country	1918 population (millions)	Number of reported deaths			
		1900–04	1905–09	1910–14	1915–19
Finland	3	295	155	182	1 605
Germany	65	165	231	136	1 323
Italy	34	18 590	2 149	8 773	17 453
Russia	134	218 000	221 000	200 000	535 000[a]

[a] Includes nonfatal cases.

The HIV epidemic is an example of an infectious disease that has become endemic in many areas, while in other areas it still causes epidemics in previously unexposed populations.[8]

In the cases of malaria and dengue fever, where mosquitoes are the vectors, the endemic areas are constrained by climate. If the area is too cold or dry and the vector cannot survive or reproduce, the disease does not become endemic. Global warming is changing the climate in some parts of the world in ways that increase the size of the endemic areas, and these vector-borne diseases are spreading to new areas.[9]

Emerging and re-emerging infections

In the last decades of the 20th century, more than 30 previously unknown or formerly well controlled communicable diseases emerged or re-emerged, with devastating consequences.[10] Of these, HIV/AIDS has had the greatest impact. The viral haemorrhagic fevers include: Ebola, Marburg, Crimean-Congo, yellow fever, West Nile and dengue. Other problematic viruses include poliomyelitis, the SARS coronavirus and influenza A. A small epidemic of new variant Creutzfeldt–Jakob disease in humans followed an epidemic of bovine spongiform encephalopathy in cattle. Among the bacterial diseases, anthrax, cholera, typhoid, plague, borelliosis, brucellosis and Buruli ulcer are proving difficult to control. Malaria leads the parasitic diseases in terms of burden, but trypanosomiasis, leishmaniasis and dracunculiasis are also defying eradication efforts. These threats to human health in the 21st century require international coordination for effective surveillance and response (Box 7.2).

While some of these emerging diseases appear to be genuinely new, others, such as viral haemorrhagic fever, may have existed for centuries yet recognized only recently because ecological or other environmental changes have increased the risk of human infection, or the ability to detect such infection has improved. This is called ascertainment bias, and is difficult to quantify. Changes in hosts, agents and environmental conditions are thought to be responsible for epidemics like the ones of diphtheria, syphilis and gonorrhea in the early 1990s in the newly independent states of eastern Europe.

Influenza pandemics arise when a novel influenza virus emerges, infects humans and spreads efficiently among them. The virus of most recent concern is the H5NI strain of influenza A (Box 7.4), one of many viruses that usually infect poultry and migratory birds. Severe influenza pandemics in 1918, 1957 and 1968 caused the deaths of tens of millions of people; for example, between 40 million and 50 million people died in the 1918 pandemic.

Box 7.2. Global Outbreak Alert and Response Network (GOARN)

The Global Outbreak Alert and Response Network (GOARN) was developed in response to SARS to deal with epidemic-prone and emerging diseases. GOARN is a collaborative framework between institutions and networks that pool human and technical resources for rapid identification, confirmation of and response to outbreaks of international importance. This network contributes to global health security by:

- combating the international spread of outbreaks;
- ensuring that appropriate technical assistance reaches affected states rapidly; and
- assisting long-term epidemic preparedness and capacity building.

All countries are obliged to report diseases of potential public health significance to WHO under the terms of the revised International Health Regulations (Box 7.3).

Box 7.3. International Health Regulations

The purpose of the International Health Regulations is to maximize protection against the international spread of diseases, while minimizing interference with world travel and trade.[11, 12]

The original International Health Regulations of 1969 were designed to control four infectious diseases: cholera, plague, yellow fever and smallpox. The revised International Health Regulations of 2005 were developed to manage public health emergencies of international concern, regardless of the particular pathogen.

The new regulations oblige countries to:

- notify WHO of all "public health emergencies of international concern";
- verify outbreaks at WHO's request;
- maintain national core capacity for early warning and response; and
- cooperate with rapid international risk assessment and assistance.

Based on projections from the 1957 pandemic, between 1 million and 4 million human deaths could occur if the H5N1 virus mutates to cause a readily transmissible form of human influenza.[13]

Chain of infection

Communicable diseases occur as a result of the interaction between:

- the infectious agent
- the transmission process
- the host
- the environment.

The control of such diseases may involve changing one or more of these components, all of which are influenced by the environment. These diseases can have a wide range of effects, varying from silent infection – with no signs or symptoms – to severe illness and death.

The major thrust of communicable disease epidemiology is to clarify the processes of infection to develop, implement and evaluate appropriate control measures. Knowledge of each factor in a chain of infection may be required before effective intervention can take place. However, this is not always necessary; it may be possible to control a disease with only a limited knowledge of its specific chain of infection. For example, improvement of the water supply in London in the 1850s prevented further cholera epidemics decades before the responsible agent was identified. However, knowledge alone is not sufficient to prevent epidemics, and cholera remains an important cause of death and disease in many parts of the world.

> **Box 7.4. Epidemiology and avian influenza**
>
> Poultry farms were affected by the highly pathogenic H5N1 virus in 2003 in Asia, and outbreaks spread to parts of Europe and Africa in 2005–06 as 40 million birds were slaughtered in an attempt to contain the spread of this virus. People are not easily infected; most of the 258 human cases confirmed by November 2006 had a history of direct and prolonged contact with infected poultry or domestic ducks.[14] However, this low transmissibility has to be seen in the context of a very high case-fatality rate: 50% of these confirmed cases died. The incubation period in humans is 2–8 days. The virus causes a high fever leading to pneumonia which does not respond to antibiotics. This virus theoretically has the potential of evolving to a form that can be spread easily between people.[15] The main strategy for addressing a potential human pandemic is to contain outbreaks in poultry as well as in humans, prevent the spread of the H5N1 virus to new countries and reduce the opportunities for human infections.[13–15]

The infectious agent

A large number of microorganisms cause disease in humans. Infection is the entry and development or multiplication of an infectious agent in the host. Infection is not equivalent to disease, as some infections do not produce clinical disease. The specific characteristics of each agent are important in determining the nature of the infection, which is determined by such factors as:

- The *pathogenicity* of the agent: its ability to produce disease, measured by the ratio of the number of persons developing clinical illness to the number exposed.
- *Virulence:* a measure of the severity of disease, which can vary from very low to very high. Once a virus has been attenuated in a laboratory and is of low virulence, it can be used for immunization, as with the poliomyelitis virus.
- *Infective dose:* the amount required to cause infection in susceptible subjects.

- *The reservoir* of an agent: its natural habitat, which may include humans, animals and environmental sources.
- *The source* of infection: the person or object from which the host acquires the agent. Knowledge of both the reservoir and the source is necessary if effective control measures are to be developed. An important source of infection may be a carrier – an infected person who shows no evidence of clinical disease. The duration of the carrier state varies between agents. Carriers can be asymptomatic throughout the course of infection or the carrier state may be limited to a particular phase of the disease. Carriers played a large role in the worldwide spread of the human immunodeficiency virus due to inadvertent sexual transmission during the long asymptomatic period.

Transmission

The second link in the chain of infection is the transmission or spread of an infectious agent through the environment or to another person. Transmission may be direct or indirect (Table 7.2).

Table 7.2. Modes of transmission of an infectious agent

Direct transmission	Indirect transmission
Touching Kissing	Vehicle-borne (contaminated food, water, towels, farm tools, etc.)
Sexual intercourse	Vector-borne (insects, animals)
Other contact (e.g. childbirth, medical procedures, injection of drugs, breastfeeding)	Airborne, long-distance (dust, droplets) Parenteral (injections with contaminated syringes)
Airborne, short-distance (via droplets, coughing, sneezing)	
Transfusion (blood)	
Transplacental	

Direct transmission
Direct transmission is the immediate transfer of the infectious agent from an infected host or reservoir to an appropriate entry point through which human infection can take place. This may be by direct contact such as touching, kissing or sexual intercourse, or by the direct spread of droplets by sneezing or coughing. Blood transfusions and transplacental infection from mother to fetus are other important means of direct transmission.

Indirect transmission
Indirect transmission may be vehicle-borne, vector-borne or airborne. Vehicle-borne transmission occurs through contaminated materials such as food, clothes, bedding and cooking utensils. Vector-borne transmission occurs when the agent is carried by an insect or animal (the vector) to a susceptible host; the agent may or may not multiply in the vector. Long-distance airborne transmission occurs when there is dissemination of very small droplets to a suitable point of entry, usually the respiratory tract. Dust particles also facilitate airborne transmission, for example, of fungal spores.

It is important to distinguish between types of transmission when selecting control methods. Direct transmission can be interrupted by preventing contact with the source; indirect transmission requires different approaches, such as the provision of mosquito nets, adequate ventilation, cold storage for foods or sterile syringes and needles.

Host

The host is the third link in the chain of infection and is defined as the person or animal that provides a suitable place for an infectious agent to grow and multiply under natural conditions. The points of entry to the host vary with the agent and include the skin, mucous membranes, and the respiratory and gastrointestinal tracts.

The reaction of the host to infection is extremely variable, being determined by the interaction between host, agent and mode of transmission. The spectrum of this reaction ranges from no apparent signs or symptoms to severe clinical illness, with all possible variations between these two extremes. The incubation period—the time between entry of the infectious agent and the appearance of the first sign or symptom of the disease—varies from a few hours (staphylococcal food poisoning) to years (AIDS).

The consequences of infection are largely determined by the host's resistance. Such resistance is usually acquired through previous exposure to or immunization against the agent in question. Immunization (or vaccination) is the protection of susceptible individuals from communicable disease by the administration of a vaccine, which can be:

- a living modified infectious agent (as for measles)
- inactivated organisms (as for pertussis)
- an inactive toxin (as for tetanus)
- bacterial polysaccharides.

Antibodies – which are formed as part of the natural immune response to pathogens – can be pooled from blood donations and given as post-exposure prophylaxis for a few diseases (such as rabies, diphtheria, varicella-zoster and hepatitis B) to people that have not been adequately immunized. This is called passive immunization, and is done on a much smaller scale than active immunization due to its risks, indications and cost. Passive transmission of maternal antibodies through the placenta can also confer resistance to infection in the fetus.

Environment

The environment plays a critical role in the development of communicable diseases. General sanitation, temperature, air pollution and water quality are among the factors that influence all stages in the chain of infection (see Chapter 9). In addition, socioeconomic factors – such as population density, overcrowding and poverty – are of great importance.

Investigation and control of epidemics

The purpose of investigating a communicable disease epidemic is to identify its cause and the best means to control it. This requires detailed and systematic epidemiological work, in the following sequential or simultaneous steps:

- undertaking preliminary investigation
- identifying and notifying cases
- collecting and analysing data
- managing and controlling
- disseminating findings and follow-up.

Investigation

The initial stage of investigation should verify the diagnoses of suspected cases and confirm that an epidemic exists. The preliminary investigation also leads to the formulation of hypotheses about the source and spread of the disease, and this in turn may lead to immediate control measures. Early reports of a possible epidemic may be based on observations made by a small number of health workers or may reflect figures gathered by the formal communicable disease notification system that operates in most countries. Sometimes reports from several health districts are needed; the number of cases in a single area may be too small to draw attention to an epidemic.

Identifying cases

The investigation of a suspected epidemic requires that new cases be systematically identified, and this means that what constitutes a case must be clearly defined (see Chapter 2). Often, detailed information on at least a sample of the cases needs to be collected. The cases reported early in an epidemic are often only a small proportion of the total; a thorough count of all cases is necessary to permit a full description of the extent of the epidemic. As soon as an epidemic is confirmed, the first priority is to control it. In severe contagious epidemics, it is often necessary to follow up contacts of reported cases to ensure the identification of all cases and limit the spread of the disease.

Management and control

The management of an epidemic involves treating the cases, preventing further spread of the disease and monitoring the effects of control measures. Treatment is straightforward except in large-scale epidemics – especially when these occur as a result of social or environmental disruption – for which external resources may be needed. The public health action required in emergencies caused by epidemics of different diseases has been described in detail.[16]

Control measures can be directed against the source and spread of infection and towards protecting people exposed to it. Usually all of these approaches are required. In some cases, however, removing the source of infection may be all that is necessary, as when a contaminated food is withdrawn from sale. An essential component of control measures is to inform health professionals and the public of the likely causes, the risk of contracting the disease and the essential control steps. This is particularly important if exposed people need to be protected through immunization, for example in containing an outbreak of measles (Box 7.5)

Once control measures have been implemented, surveillance must continue to ensure their acceptability and effectiveness. This may be relatively easy in short-term epidemics but difficult when dealing with longer-term epidemics. For example, epidemic meningococcal meningitis requires large-scale immunization programmes. Follow-up epidemiological and laboratory studies are often indicated, particularly to establish long-term cost-effectiveness.

Management and control efforts in the HIV epidemic have had some effect. Since the first cases were identified, a key approach to primary prevention has been promoting the use of condoms for prevention of HIV transmission.

> **Box 7.5. Immunization: key to prevention and control**
>
> Immunization is a powerful tool in the management and control of infectious diseases. Systematic immunization programmes can be very effective. For example, by the late 1980s, most countries in South and Latin America had incorporated measles vaccination into routine immunization programs and many had done follow-up immunization campaigns to reach all children and interrupt measles transmission.[17]

Likewise, needle exchange programs for intravenous drug users have been used successfully to limit the spread of HIV and hepatitis B virus. Education programs to make people aware of how HIV is transmitted and what they can do to prevent its spread are an essential part of primary prevention.

The HIV epidemic may have peaked in some African countries and in India. Incidence (new infections) of HIV apparently peaked in Kenya in the early to mid-1990s.[18] Because of the latency between HIV infection and death, prevalence continued to rise as incidence fell, peaking around 1997 when mortality rose to match incidence. HIV prevalence (the rate of existing infections) has also declined in south India. This reversal in trends can be partly attributed to intervention efforts that aim to decrease the number of concurrent sexual partners and increase effective use of condoms.

Surveillance and response

Definition
Health surveillance is the ongoing systematic collection, analysis and interpretation of health data essential for planning, implementing and evaluating public health activities. Surveillance needs to be linked to timely dissemination of the data, so that effective action can be taken to prevent disease. Surveillance mechanisms include compulsory notification regarding specific diseases, specific disease registries (population-based or hospital-based), continuous or repeated population surveys and aggregate data that show trends of consumption patterns and economic activity.

The scope of surveillance
The scope of surveillance is broad, from early warning systems for rapid response in the case of communicable diseases, to planned response in the case of chronic diseases which generally have a longer lag time between exposure and disease. Most countries have regulations for mandatory reporting of a list of diseases. These lists of notifiable diseases often include vaccine-preventable diseases such as polio, measles, tetanus and diphtheria as well as other communicable diseases such as tuberculosis, hepatitis, meningitis and leprosy. Reporting may be required also for

non-communicable conditions, such as maternal deaths, injuries and occupational and environmental diseases such as pesticide poisoning. Mandatory reporting of specific conditions is a subset of surveillance. There are many other uses of surveillance (Box 7.6).

Box 7.6. Uses of surveillance

Surveillance is an essential feature of epidemiologic practice and may be used to:

- recognize isolated or clustered cases;
- assess the public health impact of events and assess trends;
- measure the causal factors of disease;
- monitor effectiveness and evaluate the impact of prevention and control measures, intervention strategies and health policy changes: and
- plan and provide care.

In addition to estimating the magnitude of an epidemic and monitoring its trends, data can also be used to:

- strengthen commitment,
- mobilize communities, and
- advocate for sufficient resources.[19]

Principles of surveillance

A key principle is to include only conditions for which surveillance can effectively lead to prevention. Another important principle is that surveillance systems should reflect the overall disease burden of the community. Other criteria for selecting diseases include:

- incidence and prevalence
- indices of severity (case-fatality ratio)
- mortality rate and premature mortality
- an index of lost productivity (bed-disability days)
- medical costs
- preventability
- epidemic potential
- information gaps on new diseases.

Sources of data

Sources of data may be general or disease-specific, and include the following:

- mortality and morbidity reports
- hospital records
- laboratory diagnoses
- outbreak reports
- vaccine utilization
- sickness absence records
- biological changes in agent, vectors, or reservoirs
- blood banks.

Surveillance can collect data on any element of the causal chain of disease – behavioural risk factors, preventive actions, cases and program or treatment costs. The scope of a surveillance system is constrained by human and financial resources.

Surveillance in practice

Surveillance relies upon a routine system of reporting suspected cases within the health system, followed by validation and confirmation. Active and appropriate responses ranging from local containment measures to investigation and containment by a highly specialized team, are then put in place.

Surveillance requires continuing scrutiny of all aspects of the occurrence and spread of disease, generally using methods distinguished by their practicability, uniformity and, frequently, their rapidity, rather than by complete accuracy. The analysis of data from a surveillance system indicates whether there has been a significant increase in the reported number of cases. In many countries, unfortunately, surveillance systems are inadequate, particularly if they depend on voluntary notification.

A wide range of networks, including nongovernmental organizations, electronic discussion groups, search engines on the World Wide Web, and laboratory and training networks, offer powerful ways of obtaining information that leads to a coordinated international response.

Sentinel health information systems, in which a limited number of general practitioners report on a defined list of carefully chosen topics that may be changed from time to time, are increasingly used to provide supplementary information for the surveillance of both communicable and chronic diseases. Surveillance of chronic disease risk factors is discussed in Chapter 2. A sentinel network keeps a watchful eye on a sample of the population by supplying regular, standardized reports on specific diseases and procedures in primary health care. Regular feedback of information occurs and the participants usually have a permanent link with researchers.

Analysis and interpretation of surveillance data

Surveillance is not only a matter of collecting data, as the analysis, dissemination and use of the data for prevention and control are equally important. Many public health programs have far more data than they can presently analyse (Box 7.7).

Table 7.3 outlines Millennium Development Goal 6, which focuses on HIV/AIDS, malaria and "other diseases," which are largely interpreted as communicable diseases. Non-communicable diseases – which account for the bulk of death and disability in most countries – have been omitted.

The indicators, operational definitions and overall objectives to be met for tuberculosis (target 8) are also shown in Table 7.3; all require detailed surveillance.

Box 7.7. Tuberculosis and use of surveillance data

Tuberculosis (TB) is an important re-emerging communicable disease, and TB programs are rich in data. Routine surveillance is relatively good (compared with other health problems) because TB is a life-threatening disease mostly of adults, who therefore seek help from medical practitioners who keep patient records. Moreover, treatment is usually done under supervision, so there is a great deal of information about treatment outcomes. Some of this information remains as raw data; other important data are not compiled centrally. In many countries, surveillance data are supplemented by information from population-based surveys, and the two kinds of data can be used to reinforce each other.

Analysis of routine surveillance data can determine such things as:

- national TB burden
- current trends in TB incidence
- consistency of case detection rates
- regional variations in TB incidence.

Such surveillance and analysis are needed to measure progress towards the disease-specific targets of the Millennium Development Goals (Box 7.8).

Table 7.3. Millennium Development Goal 6: Combat HIV/AIDS, malaria and other diseases

Target 8	TB indicators (23 and 24 of 48)	Proposed operational definitions	Measurable objectives
Have halted by 2015 and begun to reverse the incidence of malaria and other major diseases	TB prevalence and death rate; proportion of TB cases detected and cured under DOTS	Number of smear-positive cases (per 100 000 population); number of TB (all forms) deaths/100 000 population/year; proportion of all estimated new smear-positive TB cases detected under DOTS in a given year; proportion of registered smear-positive TB cases successfully treated under DOTS	By 2015, reduce prevalence to 50% of the year 2000 estimate; by 2015, reduce death rate to 50% of the year 2000 estimate; by 2005, reach 70% case detection; by 2005, reach 85% treatment success

Box 7.8. Millennium Development Goals (MDGs)

United Nations Member States unanimously adopted the Millennium Declaration in September 2000, setting 2015 as the year by which these overall development goals should be achieved. Eight MDGs were established as part of the road map for implementing the Millennium Declaration. These goals concern poverty and hunger, education, gender in-equality, child mortality, maternal mortality, HIV/AIDS and other major communicable diseases, environmental sustainability, and the need for global partnership in development (see http://millenniumindicators.un.org/unsd/mi/mi_goals.asp for specific goals, targets, and indicators).

While only three goals are explicitly health-focused, all have strong links to health. The MDGs emphasize reciprocal obligations between high-income and low- and middle-income countries.[20] They hold to account the authorities responsible for providing health services, and they help define the role of health in development. By setting quantitative targets and encouraging steady monitoring of progress, the MDGs maintain awareness of the urgent need for action. One of the challenges raised by the MDGs is measuring progress. Sound epidemiological information is essential for tracking progress, evaluating impact and attributing changes to different interventions, as well as for guiding decisions on program scope and focus.

Factors that influence effectiveness of surveillance systems are listed in Table 7.4.

Table 7.4. Factors that influence effectiveness of surveillance systems

Factor or element	Effective	Ineffective
Number of conditions	Fewer	Too many
Amount of information per case	Little	Too much
Burden on reporter	Small	Too complex and burdensome
Decision-makers' interest in surveillance data	High	Low
Goals for surveillance	Clear and supported	May never have been clear
Reporting strategy for serious but common conditions	Enough information to meet goals and make decisions	Complete reporting
Usefulness of data locally	High	Low
Use is limited to analysis of data and archiving	Data are well used	Limited use of data
Usefulness to decision-makers for prevention action	High	Low

Study questions

7.1   The contribution of infectious disease to total mortality in Brazil during the period 1930–2005 is shown in Figure 6.3. What possible explanations are there for the change observed?

7.2   If you were a district health officer, how would you monitor the occurrence of measles and detect an epidemic in your district?

7.3 Describe the chain of infection for foodborne disease caused by salmonella.

7.4 Comment on the obstacles that might limit the usefulness of the revised International Health Regulations.

7.5 Using tuberculosis as an example, describe the four levels of prevention outlined in Chapter 6 and actions required at each level for an appropriate and comprehensive preventive program.

References

1. *World Health Statistics 2006.* Geneva, World Health Organization, 2006.

2. Jamison DT, Breamn JG, Measham AR, Alleyne G, Claeson M, Evans DB, et al. *Disease control priorities in developing countries.* New York, Oxford University Press, pp. 817-832.

3. Gottlieb MS, Schroff R, Schanker HM, Weisman JD, Fan PT, Wolf RA, et al. *Pneumocystis carinii* pneumonia and mucosal candidiasis in previously healthy homosexual men: evidence of a new acquired cellular immunodeficiency. *N Engl J Med* 1981;305:1425-31.

4. Biggar RJ, Nasca PC, Burnett WS. AIDS-related Kaposi's sarcoma in New York City in 1977. *N Engl J Med* 1988;318:252.

5. Olsen J, Saracci R, Trichopoulos D, eds. *Teaching epidemiology.* Oxford, Oxford University Press, 2001.

6. Snow J. *On the mode of communication of cholera.* London, Churchill, 1855 (Reprinted in *Snow on cholera: a reprint of two papers.* New York, Hafner Publishing Company, 1965).

7. SARS. *How a global epidemic was stopped.* Manila, World Health Organization Regional Office for the Western Pacific, 2006.

8. Heymann D. Infectious Diseases. In: Detels R, Mcewen J, Beaglehole R, Tanaka K. *Oxford Textbook of Public Health.* Oxford, Oxford University Press, 2005.

9. McMichael AJ, Campbell-Lendrum DH, Corvalan CF, Ebi KL, Githeko AK, Scheraga JD, et al. *Climate change and human health, risks and responses.* Geneva, World Health Organization, 2003.

10. *Report on infectious diseases: removing obstacles to health development.* Geneva, World Health Organization, 1999.

11. *International Health Regulations 2005.* Geneva, World Health Organization, 2006.

12. Baker MG, Fidler D. Global public health surveillance under new international health regulations. *Emerg Inf Dis* 2006;12:1058-65.

13. *Avian influenza: assessing the pandemic threat.* WHO/CDS/2005.29. Geneva, World Health Organization, 2005.

14. Epidemiology of WHO-confirmed cases of avian influenza A (H5N1) infection. *Wkly Epidemiol Rec* 2006;81:249-60.

15. Ungchusak K, Auewarakul P, Dowell SF, Kitphati R, Auwanit W, Puthavathana P, et al. Probable person-to-person transmission of avian influenza A (H5N1). *N Engl J Med* 2005;352:333-40.

16. Bres P. *Public health action in emergencies caused by epidemics: a practical guide.* Geneva, World Health Organization, 1986.

17. de Quadros CA. Can measles be eradicated globally? *Bull World Health Organ* 2004;82:134-8.

18. Shelton JD, Halperin DT, Wilson D. Has global HIV incidence peaked? *Lancet* 2006;367:1120-2.

19. Rehle T, Lazzari S, Dallabetta G, Asamoah-Odei E. Second-generation HIV surveillance: better data for decision-making. *Bull World Health Organ* 2004;82:121-7.

20. Haines A, Cassels A. Can the Millenium Development Goals be attained? *BMJ* 2004;329:394-7.

Chapter 8
Clinical epidemiology

Key messages

- Clinical epidemiology is the application of epidemiological principles and methods to the practice of medicine.
- With rising health-care costs, clinical practice has become a common subject of epidemiological research.
- Evidence-based guidelines have improved clinical outcomes.
- However, effective treatments are not fully used, and ineffective or costly and unnecessary treatments are still being prescribed.

Introduction

Clinical epidemiology is the application of epidemiological principles and methods to the practice of clinical medicine. It usually involves a study conducted in a clinical setting, most often by clinicians, with patients as the subjects of study. The discipline refines methods developed in epidemiology and integrates them with the science of clinical medicine. The aim of clinical epidemiology is to aid decision-making about identified cases of disease. Clinical epidemiology – which includes the methods used by clinicians to audit the processes and outcomes of their work – is a basic medical science.

Because epidemiology deals with populations and clinical medicine deals with individuals, it has been suggested that clinical epidemiology is a contradiction in terms. However, clinical epidemiology is simply concerned with a defined patient population rather than the usual community-based population.

The central concerns of clinical epidemiology are:

- definitions of normality and abnormality
- accuracy of diagnostic tests
- natural history and prognosis of disease
- effectiveness of treatment and
- prevention in clinical practice.

Definitions of normality and abnormality

The first priority in any clinical consultation is to determine whether the patient's symptoms, signs or diagnostic test results are normal or abnormal. This is necessary before any further investigations or treatment. It would be easy if a clear distinction could always be made between measurements of normal and abnormal people. Regrettably, this is rarely the case, except in genetic disorders determined by a single dominant gene. Measurements of health-related variables can be expressed as frequency distributions in the population of patients. Occasionally the frequency distributions for abnormal and normal measurements are quite different, but more often there is only one distribution and the so-called abnormal people are at the tail end of the normal distribution (see Chapter 4). There are three ways of distinguishing results in such a distribution:

- normal as common
- abnormal as associated with disease
- abnormal as treatable.

Normal as common

This definition classifies values that occur frequently as normal and those that occur infrequently as abnormal. We assume that an arbitrary cut-off point on the frequency distribution (often two standard deviations above or below the mean) is the limit of normality and consider all values beyond this point abnormal. This is called an operational definition of abnormality. If the distribution is in fact Gaussian (normal in the statistical sense), we would identify 2.5% of the population as abnormal by using this cut-off. An alternative approach, which does not assume a statistically normal distribution, is to use percentiles: we can consider that the 95th percentile point is the dividing line between normal and abnormal, thus classifying 5% of the population as abnormal (see Chapter 4).

However, there is no biological basis for using an arbitrary cut-off point as a definition of abnormality for most variables. For example, there is a continuous association between systolic blood pressure and cardiovascular disease (Figure 8.1).

Figure 8.1. Associations between blood pressure and heart disease and stroke[1]

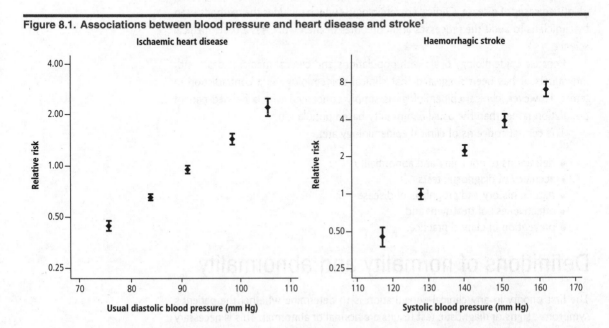

Even within the normal ranges, as determined statistically, there is an increased risk of disease compared with lower levels. Risk is a graded process; there is no cut-off point at which risk suddenly begins to increase. Most deaths from coronary heart disease happen in people who have serum cholesterol levels in the middle of the population range; only a small proportion of deaths occur in people who have very high serum cholesterol levels.

Abnormality associated with disease

Our second option is based on the distribution of the measurements for both healthy and diseased people, and we can attempt to define a cut-off point that clearly separates the two groups. A comparison of two frequency distributions often shows considerable overlap – as illustrated by serum cholesterol distributions for people with and without coronary heart disease. Choosing a cut-off point that neatly separates cases from non-cases is clearly impossible (see Figure 6.7). There are always some healthy people on the abnormal side of the cut-off point, and some true cases on the normal side.

These two types of classification error can be expressed quantitatively in terms of the sensitivity and specificity of a test, as discussed in Chapter 6.

- Sensitivity is the proportion of truly diseased people who are categorized as abnormal by the test.
- Specificity is the proportion of truly normal people categorized as normal by the test. A balance always has to be struck between sensitivity and specificity; increasing one reduces the other.

Abnormal as treatable

These difficulties in distinguishing accurately between normal and abnormal have led to the use of criteria determined by evidence from randomized controlled trials, which can be designed to detect the point at which treatment does more good than harm. Unfortunately, many treatment decisions have to be made in the absence of such evidence.

The treatment of high blood pressure is a good example – early clinical trials provided firm evidence that treating very high diastolic blood pressure ($\geq$ 120mmHg) was beneficial. Subsequent trials have indicated that the benefits of treatment outweigh the problems at lower levels of diastolic pressure, perhaps as low as 90mmHg.

However, such trials are usually not designed to account for other risk factors or the cost of treatment. More sophisticated cost-effectiveness studies may make it possible to factor the economic consequences of treatment into clinical decisions. We could then determine blood pressure levels at which treatment makes economic as well as medical sense for men and women in specific groups at risk. Treating a young woman with a diastolic blood pressure of 90 mmHg, who is at low overall risk of cardiovascular disease, will be much less cost-effective than treating an older man with a diastolic blood pressure of 90 mmHg, who has a much greater risk of cardiovascular disease. However, if the treatment of the young woman has no negative side-effects for her except the cost, she may choose to pay for the treatment herself.[2]

What is considered to be worth treating changes with time; Figure 8.2 shows the changing definition of treatable levels of blood pressure. As clinical trials gather new evidence, treatment recommendations tend to change.

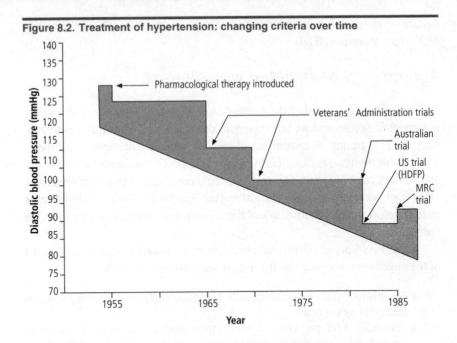

Figure 8.2. Treatment of hypertension: changing criteria over time

However, each time that a new cut-off point is proposed, we need to consider the logistic and cost implications. For example, if we take an evidence-based approach to treating people with mildly elevated blood pressure, we should be more concerned with assessing patients' absolute (or baseline) risk of cardiovascular disease, and place less emphasis on their actual blood pressure.[3] Such risk prediction can help clinicians communicate with patients (Box 8.1).

Box 8.1. Risk prediction

Risk prediction (defining absolute risk of an event over a specified time period) provides clinicians with absolute measures of the effects of treatment and assists them in helping individuals with treatment decisions. Risk prediction charts can be used to account for multiple risk factors[4]. For example, a 5-year cardiovascular disease risk – of fatal or non-fatal events – is determined largely by a person's sex, age, diabetic status, smoking history, systolic blood pressure and total cholesterol. An individual's overall cardiovascular risk can be computed from a risk prediction chart. See http://www.nzgg.org.nz/guidelines/CVD_Risk_Chart.pdf for an example.

Diagnostic tests

The first objective in a clinical situation is to diagnose any treatable disease. The purpose of diagnostic testing is to help confirm possible diagnoses suggested by the patient's signs and symptoms. While diagnostic tests usually involve laboratory investigations (genetic, microbiological, biochemical or physiological), the principles that help to determine the value of these tests should also be used to assess the diagnostic value of signs and symptoms.

Value of a test

A disease may be either present or absent and a test result either positive or negative. There are thus four possible combinations of disease status and test result, as shown in Figure 8.3 and described in relation to screening tests in Chapter 6.

In two of these combinations the test has given correct answers (true positive and true negative), and in the other two situations it has given wrong answers (false positive and false negative). We can only use these categories when there is an absolutely accurate method of determining the presence or absence of disease, against which the we can determine the accuracy of other tests. Rarely is such a method available, particularly where chronic noncommunicable diseases are concerned. For this reason, and because wholly accurate tests are likely to be expensive and invasive, simpler and cheaper tests are used in routine clinical practice. Even then, we still need to know and account for the validity, accuracy and precision of these tests when interpreting the results.

Figure 8.3. Relationship between a diagnostic test result and the occurrence of disease

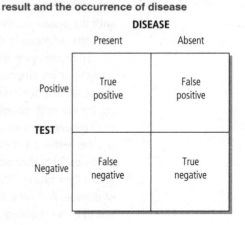

To determine the practical utility of a given test, we need to know more about how it performs. A test's positive and negative predictive value are particularly important. The positive predictive value is the probability of disease in a patient with an abnormal test result, while the negative predictive value is the probability of a patient not having a disease when the test result is negative.

Predictive value depends on the sensitivity and specificity of the test and, most importantly, on the prevalence of the disease in the population being tested. Even with a high sensitivity and high specificity (Chapter 6), if the prevalence is low the positive predictive value of a test may be very low. The predictive values of a test in clinical practice depend critically on the prevalence of the abnormality in the patients being tested; this may well differ from the prevalence in a published study on the usefulness of the test.[5]

Natural history and prognosis

The term natural history refers to the stages of a disease, which include:

- pathological onset;
- the presymptomatic stage, from onset of pathological changes to the first appearance of symptoms or signs; and
- the stage when the disease is clinically obvious and may be subject to remissions and relapses, regress spontaneously or progress to death.

Detection and treatment at any stage can alter the natural history of a disease, but the effects of treatment can only be determined if the natural history of the disease in the absence of treatment is known.

Prognosis

Prognosis is the prediction of the course of a disease and is expressed as the probability that a particular event will occur in the future. Predictions are based on defined groups of patients, and the outcome may be quite different for individual patients.

However, knowledge of the likely prognosis is helpful in determining the most useful treatment. Prognostic factors are characteristics associated with outcome in patients with the disease in question. For example, in a patient with acute myocardial infarction, the prognosis is directly related to residual heart muscle function.

Epidemiological information from many patients is necessary to provide sound predictions on prognosis and outcome. Clinical experience alone is inadequate for this purpose, since it is often based on a limited set of patients and inadequate follow-up. For example, patients who are seen by a doctor are not necessarily representative of all patients with a particular disease. Patients may be selected according to severity or other features of their disease, or by demographic, social or personal characteristics of the patients themselves. Furthermore, since many doctors do not systematically follow their patients, they have a limited, and often pessimistic, view of the prognosis of disease. A clinical observation of improved prognosis over time can be real and due to better treatment, but it can also be an artefact because of an increase in milder cases receiving treatment. Properly designed epidemiological research can produce reliable information about prognosis.

Quality of life

Ideally, the assessment of prognosis should include measurement of all clinically relevant outcomes and not just death, since patients are usually as interested in the quality of life as they are in its duration. In studies to determine natural history and prognosis, the group of patients should be randomly selected; otherwise selection bias may compromise the quality of information obtained. For example, the prognosis of patients with chest pain admitted to hospital is likely to be worse than that of patients with chest pain seen by health workers in the community.

Quantity of life

Prognosis in terms of mortality is measured as case-fatality rate or probability of survival. Both the date of onset and the duration of follow-up must be clearly specified. Survival analysis is a simple method of measuring prognosis. The pattern of survival following acute myocardial infarction is shown in Figure 8.4. Survival analyses may include selected groups, such as patients who survive the initial month after an event. Significantly more people in the later cohort (1991–92) survived three years after a myocardial infarction than did their counterparts 10 years earlier, which suggests improvement in secondary prevention of coronary heart disease.[6]

Life-table analysis is a more sophisticated method that attempts to predict the onset of events over time from previous patterns for all patients at risk. In the follow-up of cohorts to determine prognosis, bias is often introduced by the initial selection strategy and incomplete follow-up.

Figure 8.4. Survival following myocardial infarction (having survived 28 days from the event), Auckland, 1983–84, 1987–88, 1991–92[6]

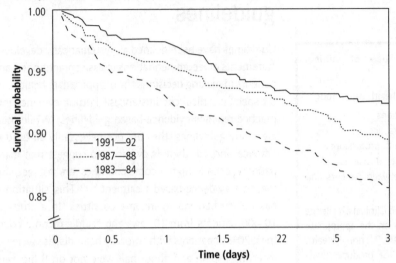

Effectiveness of treatment

Some treatments are so clearly advantageous that they require no formal assessment of indication; this is true of antibiotics for pneumonia and surgery for trauma.

However, such clarity is relatively rare in clinical medicine. Usually the effects of treatment are less obvious, and most interventions require research to establish their value. Specific treatments need be shown to do more good than harm among patients who actually use them: this is called efficacy. Treatments should also do more good than harm in all patients to whom they are offered: as not everyone will actually take what they have been prescribed, it is important to factor in the consequences of not having taken the treatment in question (Box 8.2).

In studies of efficacy it is advantageous to include only patients who are likely to be compliant. *Compliance* is the extent to which patients follow medical advice. Practical effectiveness is determined by studying outcomes in a group of people offered treatment, only some of whom will be compliant.

The best method for measuring efficacy and effectiveness is by randomized controlled trial, as described in Chapter 3. However, there are many situations in which such trials cannot be done, and only a small proportion of current medical interventions have been assessed by such trials. The growing number of well-designed trials make it possible for clinical guidelines to be based on the best available evidence (Box 8.3). Costs are often incorporated into the development of such guidelines.

Box 8.2. More good than harm?

The benefits of aspirin for patients with existing cardiovascular disease are well established, but the role of aspirin is less clear in primary prevention, especially in women. Even so, some guidelines for clinicians recommend use of low-dose aspirin in women whose 10-year risk of a first coronary event exceeds 20%. However, a meta-analysis of six relevant randomized controlled trials, which involved 51 342 women (and 44 114 men) with a low risk of a cardiovascular event who were followed up over an average of 6.4 years, found that there was no significant effect on either coronary heart disease or cardiovascular mortality, although the risk of stroke was reduced by 17% (odds ratio:0.83; 95% confidence interval: 0.70–0.97). At the same time, aspirin significantly increased the risk of major bleeding (OR: 1.68; 95% CI: 1.13–2.52).[7]

Use of evidence-based guidelines

Guidelines have been defined as systematically developed statements or recommendations to assist practitioners and patients in making decisions about appropriate health care for specific clinical circumstances.[8] Putting evidence into practice requires evidence-based guidelines. While there are many guidelines, they are not necessarily all used in practice. Indeed, there is evidence to suggest that many patients, even in high-income countries, are not receiving the best evidence-based treatment.[9, 10] This situation is particularly bad in low-income countries. In a study of 10 000 patients from 10 low- and middle-income countries, 20% of patients with coronary heart disease were not receiving aspirin and about half were not on β-blockers, which are cheap and widely available.[11]

Evidence-based guidelines are available for many diseases (see, for example, http://www.guideline.gov), and instructions for adapting them to specific national or local circumstances have been provided. The more specific and focused the approach to implementation, the more likely it is that practice will change in the direction recommended by the guideline. For example, simply providing information about the guideline is likely to have little impact, but linking this to workshops or training sessions and providing prompts within medical records is much more likely to change practice.[12]

It is also worth noting that many of the guidelines developed for high-income countries are unlikely to be immediately feasible in low- and middle-income countries. Specific national guidelines are essential. Guidelines can help curb practices like the sale of drugs without prescription by providers who may have financial incentives for selling certain products.[13] Up to 70% of drug expenditure may be unnecessary in some countries.

Prevention in clinical practice

Sound epidemiological knowledge encourages the practice of prevention in the context of ordinary clinical practice. Much of this prevention is at the secondary or tertiary level, but primary prevention can also be implemented on a routine basis (see Chapter 6). Paediatricians have long been involved in child immunization programmes, screening for inborn metabolic defects such as phenylketonuria, and the regular weighing of children and use of standard growth charts. Antenatal care is another good example of the integration of prevention into routine clinical practice.

Reducing risks

Doctors, dentists and other health workers are able to convince at least some of their patients to stop smoking. A controlled trial of different anti-smoking interventions in general practice showed that routine advice about tobacco use is useful, and that its effectiveness can be improved with a variety of techniques (Figure 8.5). In some countries, as many as 60% of current tobacco users reported receiving advice to quit smoking from their doctors.[15] Clinicians can improve their efforts to persuade patients to stop smoking by:

- enhancing the quality of the intervention offered
- focusing on smokers who are ready to quit
- increasing frequency of advice to patients
- linking with other tobacco-control intervention channels.

Figure 8.5. Stopping works: cumulative risk of lung cancer mortality.[14]

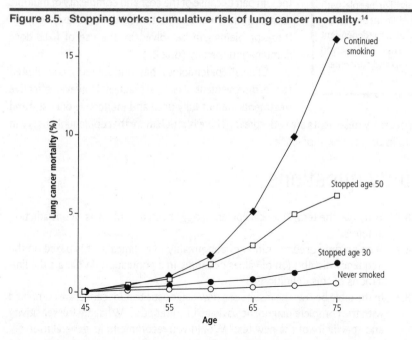

There are many other opportunities for health professionals to offer practical advice and support to patients with the hope of preventing new diseases or exacerbation of existing illnesses. Clinical epidemiologists are often involved in figuring out how effective these interventions are.

Reducing risks in patients with established disease

For cardiovascular disease and diabetes, evidence-based approaches to reducing the risk of adverse outcomes in those with the disease are very similar to the approaches used to reduce disease onset. The major difference is that the risk for future clinical events is much greater once disease is established. Both behavioural and pharmacological interventions have been shown to affect the prognosis of these diseases.

Behavioural interventions

Include promoting tobacco cessation, increased physical activity, dietary change and weight loss. Together, these may achieve a risk reduction of over 60% in people with established heart disease, and contribute to achieving good blood glucose control in people with diabetes.[16]

Box 8.4. Fixed-dose combination therapy

Fixed-dose combinations are a standard part of treatment for HIV/AIDS, tuberculosis and malaria. These have been shown to improve compliance and clinical outcomes, and to simplify distribution and storage. Likewise, a fixed-dose combination has been proposed for individuals at a high absolute risk of cardiovascular disease[17]. The components of such a polypill are off-patent and could be produced very cheaply. For people with cardiovascular disease in low- and middle-income countries, access to preventive care is usually dependent upon their ability to pay, and this large underserved group stands to gain most from a cheap and convenient formulation.

Pharmacological interventions

For people with established cardiovascular disease, international guidelines recommend long-term treatment of coagulation, high blood pressure and high cholesterol. A combination of aspirin, β-blockers, angiotensin converting enzyme inhibitors and statins is expected to reduce the risk of recurrent myocardial infarction by 75%.[17] However, there are large treatment gaps in all countries, in part because of the cost and complexity of multiple drug use and other barriers to affordable access. Some of these problems can be solved by the use of fixed-dose combination therapy (Box 8.4).

Clinical epidemiology has undoubtedly contributed to the improvement of clinical practice. However, effective treatments are not fully used and ineffective or costly and unnecessary treatments are widespread. There is much more that epidemiologists can do to improve clinical practice.

Study questions

8.1 Why has the term "clinical epidemiology" been described as a contradiction in terms?

8.2 A commonly used definition of abnormality in a clinical test is based on the frequency distribution of values occurring in a population. What are the limitations of this definition?

8.3 In the table below, the results of a new diagnostic test for cancer are compared with the complete diagnostic package in current use. What are the sensitivity and specificity of the new test? Would you recommend its general use?

8.4 What determines the positive predictive value of a screening test?

8.5 List three main advantages of randomized controlled trials in terms of helping a clinician communicate with a patient about the magnitude of a treatment effect.

8.6 The following information comes from the meta-analysis[7] of the effect of aspirin on the primary prevention of major cardiovascular events in women described in Box 8.2:

	Complete diagnosis (true disease status)	
	Disease present	Disease absent
New test Positive	8	1 000
Negative	2	9 000

- Events/total treatment group (aspirin): 682 / 25 694
- Events/total control group (placebo): 603 / 25 648
- Odds ratio (95% confidence interval): 0.88 (0.79 - 0.99)

- Relative risk reduction: RRR = (T-C/T)
- Absolute risk reduction: ARR = (T-C)
- Number needed-to-treat: NNT = (1/ARR)

Calculate the following from the above information:

a) The rate of events in the treatment group.
b) The rate of events in the control group.
c) The relative risk reduction.
d) The absolute risk reduction.
e) The number of women who would need to use low-dose aspirin to prevent 1 cardiovascular event over 6.4 years (NNT).
f) The number of women who would need to take low-dose aspirin for 1 year to prevent a cardiovascular event.
g) The average absolute benefit (or the number of cardiovascular events aspirin therapy would prevent per 1000 women).

8.7   List some of the potential limitations of the meta-analysis mentioned in the study in Box 8.2.

8.8   On the basis of this meta-analysis, what recommendations would you expect a clinician to make to concerning the use of aspirin in women?

References

1. The World Health Report. *Reducing Risks, Promoting Healthy Life.* Geneva, World Health Organization, 2002.
2. Jackson RT. Guidelines for managing raised blood pressure: Evidence based or evidence burdened? *BMJ* 1996;313:64-5.
3. Jackson R, Barham P, Bills J, Birch T, McLennan L, MacMahon S, et al. The management of raised blood pressure in New Zealand. *BMJ* 1993;307:107-10.
4. Manuel DG, Lim J, Tanuseputro P, Anderson GM, Alter DA, Laupacis A, et al. Revisiting Rose: strategies for reducing coronary heart disease. *BMJ* 2006;332:659-62.
5. Altman DG, Bland JM. Statistics Notes: Diagnostic tests 2: predictive values. *BMJ* 1994;309:102.
6. Stewart AW, Beaglehole R, Jackson R, Bingley W. Trends in 3-year survival following acute myocardial infarction 1983–92. *Eur Heart J* 1999;20:803-7.
7. Berger JS, Roncaglioni MC, Avanzini F, Pangrazzi I, Tognoni G, Brown DL. Aspirin for the primary prevention of cardiovascular events in women and men: a sex-specific meta-analysis of randomized controlled trials. *JAMA* 2006;295:306-13.
8. Field MJ, Lohr KN, eds. *Guideline for clinical practice – from development to use.* Washington, DC, National Academy Press, 1992.
9. *Guide for guidelines: a guide for clinical guideline development.* Brussels, International Diabetes Federation, 2003. (http://www.idf.org/home/index.cfm?node=1044).
10. Grimshaw J, Eccles M, Tetroe J. Implementing clinical guidelines: current evidence and future implications. *J Contin Educ Health Prof* 2004;24:S31-7.

11. Mendis S, Abegunde D, Yusuf S, Ebrahim S, Shaper G, Ghannem H, et al. WHO study on Prevention of REcurrences of Myocardial Infarction and StrokE (WHO-PREMISE) (WHO-PREMISE (Phase I) Study Group). *Bull World Health Organ* 2005;83:820-8.

12. Garg AX, Adhikari NK, Mcdonald H, Rosas-Arellano MP, Devereaux PJ, Beyene J, et al. Effects of computerized clinical decision support systems on practitioner performance and patient outcomes: a systematic review. *JAMA* 2005;293:1223-38.

13. Whitehead M, Dahlgren G, Evans T. Equity and health sector reforms: can low-income countries escape the medical poverty trap? *Lancet* 2001;358:833-6.

14. Lloyd-Jones DM, Leip EP, D'Agostino R, Beiser H, Wilson PW, Wolf PA, Levy MI. Prediction of lifetime risk for cardiovascular disease by risk factor burden at 50 years of age. *Circulation* 2006;113;791-789.

15. Jamrozik K, Vessey M, Fowler G, Wald N, Parker G, Van Vunakis H. Controlled trial of three different antismoking interventions in general practice. *BMJ* 1984;288:1499-503.

16. Murray CJ, Lauer JA, Hutubessy RC, Niessen L, Tomijima N, Rodgers A, et al. Effectiveness and costs of interventions to lower systolic blood pressure and cholesterol: a global and regional analysis on reduction of cardiovascular-disease risk. *Lancet* 2003;361:717-25.

17. Wald NJ, Law MR. A strategy to reduce cardiovascular disease by more than 80%. *BMJ* 2003;326:1419-24.

Chapter 9
Environmental and occupational epidemiology

Key messages

- The environment in which we live and work strongly influences the causation of disease and injuries.
- Exposures to environmental factors can be quantified as a "dose" which is used to establish dose-effect and dose–response relationships.
- Health impact assessments are used to forecast the likely health impact of major human interventions in the environment.
- Injury epidemiology has been used to identify which specific preventive actions are most likely to be effective.

Environment and health

The human environment consists of very basic elements: the air we breathe, the water we drink, the food we eat, the climate surrounding our bodies and the space available for our movements. In addition, we exist in a social and cultural environment, which is of great importance for our mental and physical health.

Most diseases are either caused or influenced by environmental factors. We need to understand the ways in which specific environmental factors can interfere with health to design effective prevention programmes. Environmental epidemiology provides a scientific basis for studying and interpreting the relationships between the environment and population health. Occupational epidemiology deals specifically with environmental factors in the workplace. Physical injuries are strongly dependent on factors in the living or working environment but are also strongly determined by behavioural factors. In common language the word "accident" is often applied to the events that precede an injury, but it can be misleading as the word accident implies a random event rather than a combination of predictable causal factors. In this chapter we shall use the term "environment" as a broad term for all factors external to the body that may cause disease or injury. The different environmental factors that influence health are shown in Table 9.1.[1]

The environmental and occupational health field includes a large number of specific and proximate causal factors using the concepts described for hierarchies of causes described in Chapter 5. The more distal risk factors can be analysed using the DPSEEA framework as in Figure 5.5 for transport and health. The hierarchy of causes in environmental and occupational health are shown in Box 9.1.

Impact of exposure to environmental factors

Calculations of the global burden of disease have shown how much environmental factors contribute to overall health. Between 25% and 35% of the global burden of disease may be caused by exposure to environmental factors.[2, 3] The major health problems are associated with unsafe drinking water and sanitation, indoor air pollution due to biomass energy use for cooking and heating, and urban air pollution from motor vehicles and electric power generation.[3]

High burden in low-income countries

The environmental disease burden is much higher in low-income countries than in high-income countries, although in the case of certain noncommunicable diseases, such as cardiovascular diseases and cancers, the per-capita disease burden is larger in high-income countries. Children bear the highest death toll, with more than 4 million environmentally caused deaths yearly, mostly in developing countries. The infant death rate from environmental causes is 12 times higher in low-income than in high-income countries, reflecting the human health gain that could be achieved by supporting healthy environments.[3]

Multi-causality

In epidemiological studies of environmental factors, each factor is often analysed in isolation. It should be remembered, however, that there are many ways in which environmental factors can influence each other's effects. Multi-causality and a clear hierarchy of causes (see Chapter 5) are often evident; this may explain differences between the results of observational epidemiological studies conducted in different places. How an environmental factor affects an individual also depends on other risk factor exposures and individual characteristics, such as:

- age and sex
- genetic factors
- presence of disease
- nutrition
- personality
- physical condition.

Occupational epidemiology is usually concerned with an adult population that is young or middle-aged, and often predominantly male. Furthermore, in occupational epidemiology most exposed persons are relatively healthy, at least when they start working.

Table 9.1. Environmental factors that may affect health

Factors	Examples
Psychological	Stress, unemployment, shiftwork, human relationships
Biological	Bacteria, viruses, parasites
Physical	Climate, noise, radiation, ergonomics
Accidental	Hazardous situations, speed, influence of alcohol, drugs
Chemical	Tobacco, chemicals, dust, skin irritants, food additives

Box 9.1. Hierarchy of causes in environmental and occupational health[1]

Driving forces behind current health-environment trends

- Population dynamics
- Urbanization
- Poverty and equity
- Science and technology
- Consumption and production patterns
- Economic development

Major human activities affecting environmental quality

- Household wastes
- Fresh water
- Land use and agricultural development
- Industrialization
- Energy

Poor environmental quality: exposures and risks

- Air pollution
- Food
- Soil
- Housing
- The workplace
- The global environment

In contrast, epidemiological studies of factors in the general environment would normally include children, elderly people and sick people. Exposed people in the general population are likely to be more sensitive to such factors than workers in industry. This is of great importance when the results of occupational epidemiology studies are used to establish safety standards for specific environmental hazards. For instance, the effects of lead occur at lower exposure levels in children than in adults (Table 9.2). Lead in blood is an accepted way of measuring exposure and the levels listed for the two different health outcomes are those that would most likely protect most of a population from outcomes. The level at which neurobehavioural function changes start occurring in children may be even lower than the 100 ug/l mentioned in the table.[4]

Table 9.2. Lowest blood lead levels (µg/l) at which effects on health have been reported in children and adults[5, 6]

Effect	Children	Adults
Decreased haemoglobin levels	400	500
Changes in neurobehavioural function	100	400

Evaluation of preventive measures

The main emphasis in environmental and occupational epidemiology has been on studies of the causes of disease. Specific preventive measures to reduce exposures and the impact of occupational health services also need evaluating. Exposure to hazardous environmental factors is often the result of some industrial or agricultural activity that brings economic benefit to the community, and the costs of eliminating these exposures can be considerable. However, environmental pollution is often costly in itself and may damage agricultural land or industrial property as well as people's health. Epidemiological analyses, health impact assessments and cost-effectiveness analyses help public health authorities to find an acceptable balance between health risks and the economic costs of prevention.

Value of prevention
Examples of combined epidemiological and economic analysis demonstrate the potential value of prevention.[7] In three "pollution diseases" that occurred in the 1960s in Japan, it was calculated (Table 9.2) that prevention would have been cheaper than the cure for each of the three diseases.[8] Costs included compensation of the victims and repairing environmental damage, compared with the estimated cost of pollution control to prevent the diseases. The benefit-cost ratio was 100 for mercury pollution and the resulting Minamata disease (Table 9.3).

Future challenges
Environmental epidemiology will face new challenges in the coming decades with changes in the global environment. Studies are needed of the health impacts of global climate change, depletion of the ozone layer, ultraviolet radiation, acid precipitation and aspects of population dynamics.[9] Some of the different potential health effects of climate change have not yet been documented in epidemiological studies. However, as the evidence for slow climate change is accumulating around the world, epidemiological studies are contributing new knowledge to this field.[10]

Table 9.3. Pollution damage and control costs for three disease outbreaks, Japan[8] *(¥ millions, 1989 equivalents)*

Pollution disease	Main pollutant	Pollution control costs	Pollution damage costs			
			Health damage	Livelihood damage	Environmental remediation	Total
Yokkaichi asthma	SO_2, air pollution	14 800	21 000 (1 300)[a]	—	—	21 000
Minamata disease	Mercury, water pollution	125	7 670	4 270	690	12 630
Itai-Itai disease	Cadmium, water and soil pollution	600	740	880	890	2 510

a. Based on actual compensation payments to a fraction of the population. The larger figure is what it would have cost to compensate all those affected.

As seen in Figure 9.1, the range of potential health effects is very broad and several epidemiological approaches will be needed to show evidence of the emerging health changes. The Intergovernmental Panel on Climate Change — a consortium of

Figure 9.1. How climate change affects health[10]

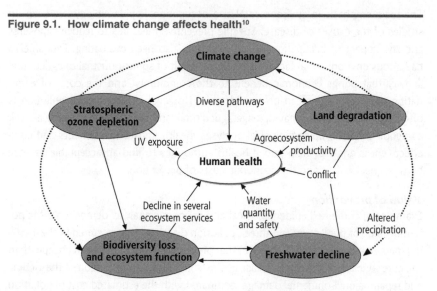

scientists coordinated by the World Meteorological Organization — publishes regular assessments of the progress of global climate change and its effects. The inputs needed from epidemiology for future research and assessments are listed in Box 9.2.[11] Epidemiologists need to document associations between climate and health outcomes for more precise and convincing evidence, and to conduct research on model scenarios. It will be necessary to account for projections and dynamics based on different climate models, and to relate climate and health with a broad range of socioeconomic environments City-specific "early warning systems" and vector-borne disease control programs are needed. Patterns of malnutrition and obesity – including food distribution and equity – also need further study.

Exposure and dose

General concepts

Epidemiological studies on the effects of environmental factors often deal with very specific factors that can be measured quantitatively. The concepts of exposure and dose are therefore particularly important in environmental and occupational epidemiology.

Exposure has two dimensions: level and duration. For environmental factors that cause acute effects more or less immediately after exposure starts, the current exposure level determines whether effects occur (for instance, the "London smog epidemic" of deaths from lung and heart disease, as shown in Figure 9.2, is one of the world's first major environmental disease outbreaks that was documented in detail).

However, many environmental factors produce effects only after a long period of exposure. This is true of chemicals that accumulate in the body (for instance,

> **Box 9.2. Epidemiological research on the health effects of climate change**
>
> Emerging large-scale risks to population health are:
> - global climate change
> - degradation of arable land
> - depletion of fisheries
> - widespread shortage of fresh water
> - losses of species and ecosystems.

Figure 9.2. The London smog epidemic,[12] December 1952

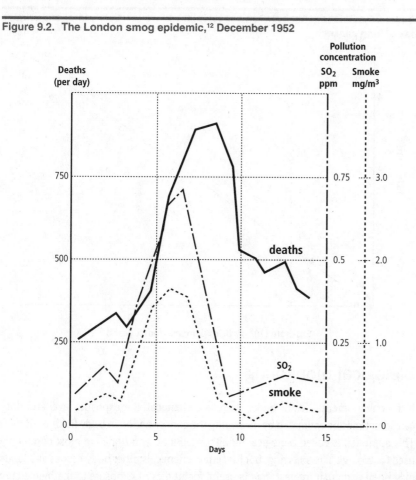

cadmium) and hazards that have a cumulative effect (for instance, radiation or noise). For these hazards, the past exposure levels and the exposure duration are more important than the current exposure level. The total exposure (or external dose) needs to be estimated. It is often approximated as the product of exposure duration and exposure level.

In epidemiological studies, all kinds of estimates of exposure and dose have been used to quantify the relationship between an environmental factor and the health status of a population. For example, in Figure 1.1, the exposure is expressed in terms of exposure level only (number of cigarettes smoked per day). Table 5.2 shows the combined effect of duration and exposure level on noise-induced hearing loss. The external dose can also be expressed as one combined measure, as with pack-years for cigarette smoking and fibre-years (or particle-years) for asbestos exposure in the workplace (Figure 9.3). Sometimes a proxy measure of exposure is used, such as the traffic flow per hour in a particular place or the petrol consumption per year as indicators of air pollution exposure. These variables could also be considered as "pressure" indicators in the causal hierarchy (Chapter 5). Other examples would be the use of pesticides in an area or the number of children living in houses painted with lead-containing paint.[13]

Figure 9.3. Relationship between asbestos exposure (particle-years) and relative risk of lung cancer[14]

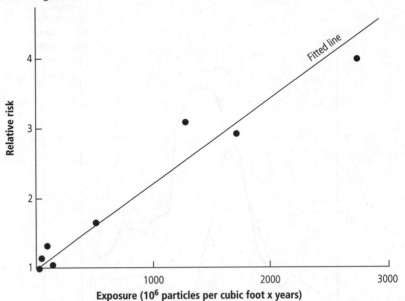

Biological monitoring

If the environmental factor under study is a chemical, the exposure level and dose can sometimes be estimated by measuring the concentration in body fluids or tissues. This approach is called biological monitoring. Blood and urine are most commonly used for biological monitoring, but for certain chemicals other body tissues and fluids may be of particular interest: hair is useful for studies of exposure to methylmercury from fish; nail clippings have been used to study arsenic exposure; analysis of faeces can give an estimate of recent exposure to metals via food (particularly lead and cadmium); breast milk is a good material for examining exposure to organochlorine pesticides and other chlorinated hydrocarbons such as polychlorinated biphenyls and dioxins; and biopsies of fat, bone, lung, liver and kidney have been used in studies of patients with suspected poisoning.

Interpreting biological data

The interpretation of biological monitoring data requires detailed knowledge of the kinetics and metabolism of chemicals, which includes data on absorption, transport, accumulation and excretion. Because of the rapid excretion of certain chemicals, only the most recent exposure to them can be measured. Sometimes one body tissue or fluid gives an indication of recent exposure and another indicates the total dose. As the chemical would have to be absorbed to reach the biological indicator material, the dose measured in this way is called the absorbed dose or internal dose, as opposed to the external dose estimated from environmental measurements.

As an example, Figure 9.4 shows the rapid increase of blood cadmium in the first months after exposure started for an industrial worker, whereas there is no apparent change in the urine cadmium level.[15] On the other hand, after long-term exposure urine cadmium is a very good indicator of the accumulated dose. One of the study questions in this chapter invites the reader to seek further specific examples.

Figure 9.4. Blood and urine levels of cadmium during the first year of occupational exposure

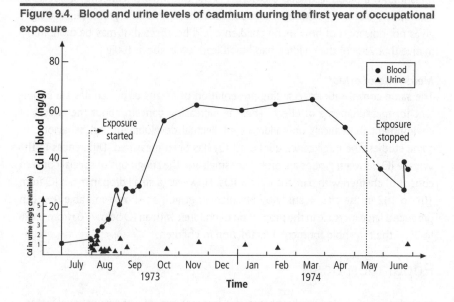

Individual versus group measurements

Variation in time
Individual measurements of exposure vary with time. The frequency of measurements and the method used to estimate the exposure or dose in an epidemiological study therefore require careful consideration. The estimate used needs to be valid (Chapter 3)

and the measurements need to be accompanied by quality assurance procedures that confirm measurement accuracy.

Variation in exposure

There is also variation in exposure or dose between individuals. Even people working side-by-side in a factory have different exposure levels because of different work habits or differences in the local distribution of a pollutant. For instance, one machine may leak fumes while another may not. If the exposure or dose is measured by biological monitoring, an additional source of variation is the difference of individual absorption and excretion rates for the chemical. Even people with the same external dose may end up with different internal doses.

Distribution issues

One way of presenting individual variations is through distribution curves (Chapter 4). The distributions of individual doses of environmental chemicals are often skewed and conform to a log-normal frequency distribution more closely than to a normal distribution. Ideally, the shape of the dose distribution should be tested in every epidemiological study where quantitative dose measurements are carried out. If the distributions are found to be log-normal, group comparisons should be carried out with geometric rather than arithmetic means and standard deviations.

Another way is to use quantiles or percentiles (see Chapter 4). For instance, in assessing whether the dose of lead in a group of children is of concern, the average may be of less interest than the proportion with individual doses above a certain threshold. If a blood lead level of 100µg/l is the threshold of concern for effects of lead on the brain, then information about the mean level in a group (e.g. 70 µg/l) gives no indication of how many children could be affected. It may be more informative that 25% of the children had blood lead levels above 100ìg/l.

Measures of effect

The same considerations regarding presentation of means or percentiles are important for measurements of effect. There is increasing concern about the effects of environmental chemicals on children's intellectual development and behaviour. In some studies, the intelligence quotient (IQ) has been measured. Differences in the average IQ between groups are often very small and the subgroups of special concern consist of children with particularly low IQs. However, a small drop in mean IQ from 107 to 102 in the classic study by Needleman et al.[16] as shown in Table 9.4, can produce a large increase in the proportion of children with an IQ below 70 (from 0.6% to 2%), the threshold for mental retardation in children.

Population dose

In epidemiological studies of cancer caused by environmental or occupational factors, another way of presenting group dose is sometimes used. This is the *dose commitment* or population dose, calculated as the sum of individual doses. For radiation, a dose commitment of 50 sievert (Sv) is expected to cause one fatal cancer. Whether the dose commitment refers to 100 people each with a dose of 0.5Sv or 10 000 people each with a dose of 5mSv, the result is one case of fatal cancer. This calculation is based on the fundamental assumptions that there is no threshold individual dose below which the cancer risk is zero and that the cancer risk increases linearly with dose. However, the dose variation within the group may be large and the people with the highest dose obviously have a higher individual cancer risk due to this environmental exposure.

Table 9.4. Full-scale and subtest scores on the Wechsler Intelligence Scale for Children (Revised) (WISC-R) for subjects with high and low lead levels in teeth[16]

WISC-R	Low lead (< 10mg/kg) (mean)	High lead (> 20mg/kg) (mean)	P-value (one-sided)
Full-scale IQ	106.6	102.1	0.03
Verbal IQ	103.9	99.3	0.03
Information	10.5	9.4	0.04
Vocabulary	11.0	10.0	0.05
Digit span	10.6	9.3	0.02
Arithmetic	10.4	10.1	0.49
Comprehension	11.0	10.2	0.08
Similarities	10.8	10.3	0.36
Performance IQ	108.7	104.9	0.08
Picture completion	12.2	11.3	0.03
Picture arrangement	11.3	10.8	0.38
Block design	11.0	10.3	0.15
Object assembly	10.9	10.6	0.54
Coding	11.0	10.9	0.90
Mazes	10.6	10.1	0.37

Dose-effect relationships

For many environmental factors, effects range from subtle physiological or biochemical changes to severe illness or death, as explained in Chapter 2. Usually, the higher the dose, the more severe or intense the effect. This relationship between *dose and severity of effect in the individual* is called the dose-effect relationship (Figure 9.5), which can be established for an individual or a group (the average dose at which each effect occurs). At a low carbon monoxide (CO) dose (measured as carboxy-haemoglobin in blood) a slight headache would be the only effect, but as the dose increases, the effects of CO become more severe as this figure shows. Not all individuals react in the same way to a given environmental exposure, so the dose-effect relationship for an individual differs from the group value.

The dose-effect relationship provides valuable information for the planning of epidemiological studies. Some effects may be easier to measure than others, and some may be of particular significance for public health. Measurements of changes in the blood or urine, so-called biomarkers, may be used to study some early subtle effects as well as the exposure. In the case of cadmium, for instance, the level of low molecular weight proteins in the urine is a good biomarker of the earliest effects on the kidney.[15] The dose-effect relationship helps the investigator choose the appropriate effect to study.

Figure 9.5. Dose-effect relationship

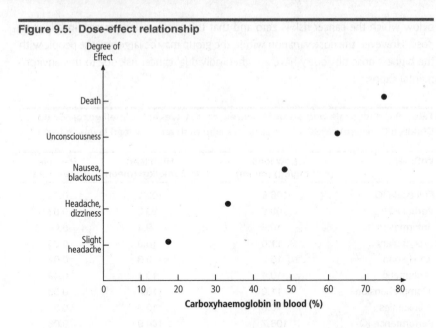

Carboxyhaemoglobin in blood (%)

In the process of establishing safety standards, the dose-effect relationship also gives useful information on effects that must be prevented and on those that may be used for screening purposes. If a safety standard is set at a level where the less severe effects are prevented, the more severe effects are also likely to be prevented, because they occur at higher doses.

Dose–response relationships

Response is defined in epidemiology as the proportion of an exposed group that develops a specific effect. Theoretically the shape of the dose–response relationship should look like an S or like a cumulative normal distribution. Many examples of dose–response relationships with this shape have been found in environmental and occupational epidemiology studies. At low doses almost nobody suffers the effect, and at a high level almost everybody does. This reflects the variation in individual sensitivity to the factor studied.

The dose–response relationship can, in some cases, be approximated to a straight-line relationship, particularly when only a narrow range of low responses is involved. This approach has been used, for instance, in the study of lung cancer risk and asbestos dose (Figure 9.3) or tobacco smoking dose (Figure 1.1). The dose–response relationship can be modified by factors such as age. This has been found, for example, for hearing loss caused by loud noise,[17] one of the most common health effects in the workplace, where a strong dose–response relationship can be demonstrated (Table 5.2). Dose–response relationships can be produced for any environmental factor where the exposure can be quantified. Examples from epidemiological studies of injuries are given in a following section.

Assessing risk

Risk assessment

Risk assessment is a term with a variety of definitions, but the intuitive interpretation is that it is some form of assessment of the health risk of a defined policy, action or intervention. WHO has produced numerous guidelines and methods for doing risk assessments, particularly in relation to chemical safety.

Health impact assessment

Health impact assessment can be considered as a risk assessment focused on a specific population or exposure situation, while risk assessment has a more general application, answering such questions as: "What type of health risk can this chemical potentially cause in certain exposure situations?" Health impact assessment is now widely recommended as a method to assess the potential value of different preventive policies and actions.[18]

Risk management

The term risk management is applied to the planning and implementation of actions to reduce or eliminate health risks.

Environmental health impact assessment

In recent years, increased attention has been given to environmental impact assessment (predictive analysis) and environmental audit (analysis of the existing situation) of industrial or agricultural development projects. These procedures have become legal requirements in many countries. The health component of these environmental assessments has been labelled environmental health impact assessment and an important application of epidemiological analysis in environmental health. Such assessment is also used to predict potential health problems in the use of new chemicals or technologies. There are several steps to assist in an overall environmental risk assessment:

Identify which environmental health hazard may be created by the technology or project under study. Are there chemical hazards? If so, which specific chemicals are involved? Are there biological hazards? (see Table 9.1).

- Analyse the type of health effect that each hazard may cause (hazard assessment). The information can be collected in systematic reviews of the scientific literature (in the same manner as a Cochrane review of treatments for specific diseases, as outlined in (Chapter 3) for each hazard or by referring to international hazard assessments, such as the Environmental Health Criteria Series or the Concise International Chemical Assessment Documents published by WHO, the Monograph Series published by the International Agency for Research on Cancer (IARC) and, if necessary, complementing this information with epidemiological studies of people exposed to the hazards in question.

- Measure or estimate the actual exposure levels for the people potentially affected, including the general population and the workforce. The human exposure assessment should take into account environmental monitoring biological monitoring and relevant information about history of exposure and changes over time.
- Combine the exposure data for subgroups of the exposed population with the dose–effect and dose–response relationships for each hazard to calculate the likely health risk in this population.

Epidemiological studies can also be used to measure health risk directly. The risk could be presented as potential increase in relative risk of certain health effects or the calculated increase in the number of cases of certain diseases or symptoms (Box 9.3).

Box 9.3. Example: health impact assessment

One example of a health impact assessment that has had major impact on environmental health policy is the assessment of the impact of traffic-related air pollution in Europe.[19] Based on air monitoring data, estimates of the number of people exposed and dose–response relationships from epidemiological studies, investigators calculated the likely number of deaths due to this type of air pollution (Table 9.5). It was striking that the number of deaths from pollution far exceeded the number of deaths from traffic accidents. This study inspired a series of policies to control traffic-related air pollution in Europe.

A similar analysis was done for New Zealand[20] with a lower ratio for air pollution deaths to traffic accident deaths (Table 9.5). This lower ratio is expected, as the air pollution levels in general are lower than in Europe and the traffic accident risks are higher.

Table 9.5. Air pollution mortality (for adults ≥ 30 years) and road death tolls (1996)

Country	Population (million)	Traffic accident deaths (A)	Mortality due to traffic air pollution (B)	Ratio B/A
France	58.3	8 919	17 629	2.0
Austria	8.1	963	2 411	2.5
Switzerland	7.1	597	1 762	3.0
New Zealand	3.7	502	399	0.8

A recent development in health impact assessments is to use burden of disease estimates in the assessments. Tools for this have been developed by WHO in the Environmental Burden of Disease document series.[21] The three key steps in risk management assessment are:

- First, estimate the health risk to be evaluated in relation to a predetermined "acceptable risk" or in relation to other health risks in the same community. Maximum exposure limits, public health targets or other policy instruments for health protection are often used in this process. The fundamental question is: is it necessary to take preventive action because the estimated health risk is too high?
- If it is decided that preventive action is needed, the next step in risk management is to reduce exposure. This may involve changing the eliminate hazards installing equipment to control pollution or moving proposed hazardous projects.
- Finally, risk management also involves monitoring of exposure and health risks after the selected controls have been put into place. It is important to ensure that the intended protection is achieved and that any additional protective measures are taken without delay. In this phase of risk management, human exposure assessments and epidemiological surveys play an important role.

Injury epidemiology

One special type of epidemiological analysis that plays an important role in environmental and occupational health is accident and injury epidemiology. Traffic accident injuries are on the increase in many countries and, being a major cause of death and disability among young people and children, they have a great impact on public health.

Dose–response relationships can also be produced for injury factors where the environmental exposure can be quantified. One example is the fatality risk of pedestrians hit by cars (Figure 9.6).

Figure 9.6. Pedestrian fatality risk as a function of the impact speed of the car[22]

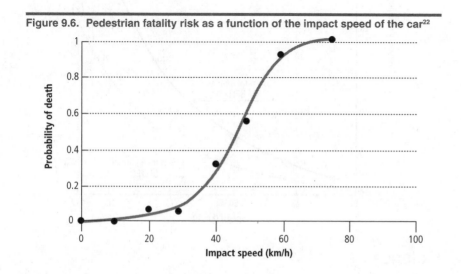

Traffic crash injuries

A classic example of practical injury epidemiology for traffic crashes is the demonstrated dose–response relationship between driving speed (dose) and frequency of injury (response) for drivers with and without seat belts (Figure 9.7). This has served as valuable information for decisions regarding two different preventive approaches: speed reduction and the use of seat-belts.

Workplace injury

Similarly, injuries are among the most important types of ill health caused by factors in the workplace. The environmental factors associated with these injuries are often more difficult to identify and quantify than those causing, for instance, chemical poisoning. However, technological and management improvements over the years have resulted in great reductions in occupational injury rates in most high-income countries (see the LABORSTA database of the International Labour Organization in Geneva).

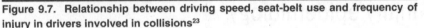

Figure 9.7. Relationship between driving speed, seat-belt use and frequency of injury in drivers involved in collisions[23]

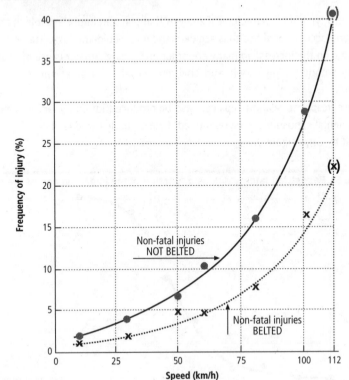

Violence

Violence is another public health problem that has been highlighted through epidemiological analysis during recent years.[24] In certain high-income countries, homicides are a major cause of death among young males, and the situation is even worse in some low- and middle-income countries. For example, the WHO mortality database shows that in Brazil, homicide accounts for 40% of all deaths among 15–24 year old males. Firearms are frequently used to commit homicide, and this is an increasing trend in several countries.

Suicides

Another important cause of death is suicide. The environmental factors causing suicidal intent are primarily social or economic,[24] but completed suicides are also dependent on access to a suicidal method, which can be seen as an environmental factor. Figure 9.8 shows the dramatic increase of suicides in Western Samoa after the introduction of the extremely toxic pesticide paraquat. It was easily available in the community because it was used on banana plantations in every village. When control measures were introduced, the incidence of suicide decreased. This is an example where simple counting of the number of incident cases can clearly show the effect of preventive interventions.

Figure 9.8. Number of suicides in Western Samoa in relation to the use of paraquat.[24]

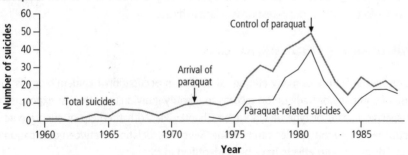

Special features of environmental and occupational epidemiology

Epidemiology is used in environmental and occupational fields to establish:

- etiology
- natural history
- the health status of a population
- the value of interventions and health services.

One special feature of environmental epidemiology is its geographic base. Air, water and soil pollution are generally related to sources with defined geographic locations. Mapping of environmental levels or exposures can therefore be useful tools in epidemiological studies.

Environmental epidemiology studies often require approximations and modeling for quantification of exposures, because individual exposure measurements are very difficult to assemble. Air quality modeling combined with geographical information system (GIS) analysis has been used in several air pollution health effect studies. One example of exposure assessment is the number of days when nitrogen dioxide concentrations exceed different cut-off points, and the number of people exposed in different parts of a city based on census data.

Setting safety standards

Dose–effect and dose–response relationships are of particular importance in environmental and occupational epidemiology because they provide the foundation for setting safety standards. The dose–effect relationship can be used to decide which effect is most important to prevent. Once a decision is made concerning an acceptable response level, the dose–response relationship gives the maximum dose that would be acceptable. WHO has developed a series of water quality guidelines,[25, 26] air quality guidelines[27] and health-based maximum occupational exposure limits[28] using this approach. In response to the accident at the Chernobyl nuclear power station, guidelines were also developed for judging the radioactive contamination of food.[29] For many environmental factors, the available data are insufficient to permit a standard to be set with any accuracy, and informed guesses or practical experience become the basis of the safety standard. Further epidemiological studies are needed to provide more information on dose–response relationships.

Measuring past exposure

One special feature of many etiological studies in occupational epidemiology is the use of company or trade union records to identify individuals with past exposure to a specific hazard or type of work (see Chapter 3). With the help of such records, retrospective cohort studies can be done. Several associations between occupational hazards and health effects have been identified in this way.

Healthy worker effect in occupational studies

Occupational epidemiology studies often include only men who are physically fit. The exposed group of workers thus has a lower overall mortality rate than the corresponding age group in the general population. The lower mortality has been called the healthy worker effect,[30] which needs to be taken into account whenever the mortality rate in a group of workers is compared with the rate in the general population. Often the rates among healthy workers are 70%–90% of those in the general population. The difference arises because of the presence of unhealthy and disabled people in the non-working population, who usually have higher mortality rates.

Continuing challenges for epidemiologists

This chapter has highlighted the significant contribution to the global burden of disease from a variety of environmental and occupational hazards. Epidemiological studies in this field have contributed essential information to health policy and prevention strategies currently applied in high-income countries. Epidemiologists now face the challenge of generating evidence of the need for similar strategies in low- and middle-income countries.

The priorities for health policy are sometimes driven by the "body count mentality", meaning that dead bodies caused by a particular health hazard have to be shown before the hazard is taken seriously. Because many environmental and occupational hazard situations are related to economic activities where cost-consciousness is high, preventive action in this area is often controversial. Epidemiology can provide a foundation for evidence-based health and environment policy.

Controversy surrounds environmental issues such as climate change – where only limited epidemiological evidence has accumulated – but action to prevent future health damage needs to be taken now. There are many opportunities for important and interesting research in occupational and environmental health, and the field is open to inventive and original approaches.

Study questions

9.1 (a) In Table 9.1, which age group is more susceptible to the effects of lead?
(b) Which effect is the more sensitive indicator of lead exposure?

9.2 (a) What is the result of the increasing external dose shown in Figure 9.3?
(b) Why are asbestos doses often calculated as particle-years or fibre-years?

9.3 Choose an environmental toxic substance and do an Internet search for potential biological monitoring materials that represent recent exposure and cumulative long-term exposure.

9.4 You are a public health official in a medium-sized city with several large industrial enterprises. The workers in these enterprises are provided with medical care through a uniform insurance system, which means that all current and retired workers are likely to get health care from the same hospital. A hospital doctor calls you and expresses concern about the large number of lung cancers among the workers. How would you design an initial study to investigate potential associations between occupational exposures and increased risk of lung cancer?

9.5 How could an epidemiological analysis of the London smog epidemic of deaths due to heart and lung disease in 1952 (Figure 9.2) ascertain that the epidemic was in fact due to smog?

9.6 What is meant by the healthy worker effect, and how can it introduce bias in occupational epidemiology studies?

9.7 Suggest study situations when GIS may be a useful tool for exposure assessment in environmental epidemiology.

9.8 Describe injury risk situations in your daily life for which preventive methods have been developed from epidemiological studies.

References

1. *Health and environment in sustainable development.* Document WHO/EHG/97.8. Geneva, World Health Organization, 1997.

2. Smith KR, Corvalan CF, Kjellstrom T. How much ill health is attributable to environmental factors? *Epidemiology* 1999;10:573-84.

3. Pruess-Ustun A, Corvalan C. *Preventing disease through healthy environments. Towards an estimate of the environmental burden of disease.* Geneva, World Health Organization, 2006.

4. Canfield RL, Henderson CR, Cory-Slechta DA, Cox C, Jusko TA, Lanphear BP. Intellectual impairment in children with blood lead concentrations below 100 ug/l. *N Engl J Med* 2003;348:1517-26.

5. Meyer PA, Pivetz T, Dignam TA, Homa DM, Schoonover J, Brody D. Surveillance for elevated blood lead levels among children in the United States, 1997–2000. *MMWR Surveill Summ* 2003;52:1-21.

6. *Inorganic lead.* (Environmental Health Criteria, No. 165).Geneva, World Health Organization, 1995.

7. Kjellström T, Lodh M, Mcmichael T, et al. Air and water pollution; burden and strategies for control. In: Jamison DT, Breamn JG, Measham AR, Alleyne G, Claeson M, Evans DB, et al, eds. *Disease control priorities in developing countries.* New York, Oxford University Press, 2006:817-832.

8. Study Group for Global Environment and Economics. Office of Planning and Research, *Pollution in Japan—Our Tragic Experience.* Tokyo, Japan Environment Agency, 1991.

9. Mcmichael AJ. *Human frontiers, environments and disease: past patterns, uncertain futures.* Cambridge, Cambridge University Press, 2001.

10. McMichael AJ, Campbell-Lendrum DH, Corvalan CF, Ebi KL, Githeko AK, Scheraga JD, et al. *Climate change and human health, risks and responses.* Geneva, World Health Organization, 2003.

11. Sunyer J, Grimault T. Global climate change, widening health inequalities and epidemics. *Int J Epidemiol* 2006;35:213-6.

12. United Kingdom Ministry of Health. *Mortality and morbidity during the London fog of December* 1952. London, Her Majesty's Stationery Office, 1954.

13. Children's health and the environment in North America. Geneva, World Health Organization.

14. Mcdonald JC, et al. Chrysolite Fibre Concentration and Lung Cancer Mortality: A Preliminary Report. In: Wagner, JC ed. *Biological Effects Of Mineral Fibres.* Vol. 2. (IARC Scientific Publications, No. 30), Lyons, International Agency for Research on Cancer, 1980:811–817.

15. *Cadmium: environmental aspects.* (Environmental health criteria No. 134). Geneva, World Health Organization, 1992.

16. Needleman HL, Gunnoe C, Leviton A, Reed R, Peresie H, Maher C, Barrett P. Deficits in psychologic and classroom performance of children with elevated dentine lead levels. *N Engl J Med* 1979;300:689-95.

17. *Noise.* (Environmental Health Criteria, No. 12). Geneva, World Health Organization, 1980.

18. Dora C, Racioppi F. Including health in transport policy agendas: the role of health impact assessment analyses and procedures in the European experience. *Bull World Health Organ* 2003;81:399-403.

19. Kunzli N, Kaiser R, Medina S, Studnicka M, Chanel O, Filliger P, et al. Public-health impact of outdoor and traffic-related air pollution: a European assessment. *Lancet* 2000;356:795-801.

20. Fisher G, Rolfe KA, Kjellstrom T, Woodward A, Hales S, Sturman AP, et al. Health effects due to motor vehicle pollution in New Zealand: Report to the Ministry of Transport. 2002:1-72.

21. *Introduction and methods - Assessing the environmental burden of disease at national and local levels.* Geneva, World Health Organization, 2003 http://www.who.int/quantifying_ehimpacts/publications/en/.

22. Peden M, Sarfiled R, Sleet D, Mohan D, Hyder AA, Jarawan E, eds. *World report on road traffic injury prevention.* Geneva, World Health Organization, 2004.

23. Bohlin NI. A statistical analysis of 28 000 accident cases with emphasis on occupant restraint value. *SAE transactions* 1967;76:2981–994.

24. Krug EG, Dahlber LL, Mercy JA, Zwi AB, Lozano R, eds. *World report on violence and health.* Geneva, World Health Organization, 2002.

25. Scoggins A, Kjellstrom T, Fisher G, Connor J, Gimson N. Spatial analysis of annual air pollution exposure and mortality. *Sci Total Environ* 2004;321:71-85.

26. *Guidelines for drinking-water quality.* Vol. 1, Recommendations. Geneva, World Health Organization, 2004.

27. *Air quality guidelines for Europe.* (Regional Publications, European Series, No. 23) Copenhagen, World Health Organization Regional Office for Europe, 1987.

28. Recommended health-based limits in occupational exposure to heavy metals: report of a WHO Study Group. *WHO Tech Rep Series* 1980;647.

29. *Derived intervention levels for radionuclides in food. Guidelines for application after widespread radioactive contamination.* Geneva, World Health Organization, 1988.

30. Mcmichael AJ. Standardized mortality ratios and the "healthy worker effect": scratching beneath the surface. *J Occup Med* 1976;18:165-8.

Chapter 10
Epidemiology, health policy and planning

Key messages

- Epidemiology informs the development, implementation, and evaluation of health policy and planning.
- Epidemiologists can be usefully involved in health policy issues.
- Techniques for assessing health policy interventions need refining.
- Health planning is a cycle that ideally incorporates continual assessment of effectiveness.

Introduction

The full value of epidemiological research is only realized when it is translated into health policy and the subsequent planning and implementation of disease or injury prevention and control programs. As we have seen, there can be a delay between the acquisition of knowledge and its uptake by health policy-makers and planners. In this chapter we describe how epidemiological knowledge informs health policy and planning. The principles remain the same through a range of activities from implementing programs to evaluating health services. But first, some definitions:

Health policy

Health policy provides a framework for health-promoting actions covering the social, economic, and environmental determinants of health. Health policy can be viewed as a set of decisions about strategic goals for the health sector and the means for achieving these goals. Policy is expressed in norms, practices, regulations and laws affecting the health of the population which together provide shape, direction and consistency to decisions made over time.

Health planning

Health service planning is a process of identifying key objectives and choosing among alternative means of achieving them. While the process implies a rational set of actions, the reality of planning is often quite unpredictable (see Box 10.5).

Evaluation

Evaluation is the process of determining – as systematically and objectively as possible – the relevance, effectiveness, efficiency and impact of activities with respect to the agreed goals. The evaluation of specific interventions is well advanced; it is much more difficult, and controversial, to determine and compare the overall performance of health systems.[1]

Epidemiologists work with other specialists to inform communities and their decision-makers so that policy choices can be made in full knowledge of the likely outcomes and costs.

Health policy

Public policy is the sum of the decisions that shape society. It provides a framework for the development of, for example, industrial and agricultural production, corporate management, and health services. It determines the range of options from which organizations and individuals make their choices, and thus directly influences the environment and patterns of living. Public policy is a major determinant of the health of the population.

Health policy is often considered in a narrow sense, referring specifically to medical care issues and the organization of health care services. However, health is influenced by a broad range of policy decisions, not just those in the medical or health field. A true health policy should therefore provide a framework for health-promoting actions covering the social, economic, and environmental determinants of health.

The influence of epidemiology

If epidemiology is intended to prevent and control disease, the results of epidemiological results must influence public policy. To date, epidemiology has not fulfilled its potential in this respect, and there are only a few areas in which epidemiological research has been fully applied. However, the importance of epidemiology in policy-making is recognized (see Box 10.1).

The influence of epidemiology is often mediated by public opinion. Policy-makers in many countries respond to public opinion rather than leading it. The growth in media attention given to epidemiological research has increased public awareness of the subject. Epidemiology is often an important factor influencing public policy but is rarely the only influence.

A major difficulty in applying epidemiology to public policy is the necessity for making judgements about the cause of a disease and decisions on what to do when the evidence is incomplete. Some epidemiologists believe their role should be limited to epidemiological research, while others consider they should be directly involved in the application of the results to public policy. This difference reflects personal, social and cultural preferences. If a health issue is controversial – and most are – epidemiologists who are involved in the public policy arena may be accused of

---

Box 10.1. Success factors in policy formulation[2]

Successful policy formulation necessitates:

- a high-level political mandate to develop a national policy framework;
- a core group of scientists who estimate health needs, advocate for action, and develop a national policy and plan;
- international collaboration providing political and technical support;
- wide consultation when drafting, reviewing, and re-drafting the policy until it is endorsed;
- awareness that the process of consultation may be as important as the content in generating support and ownership;
- development and implementation of a consistent communication strategy for all stages of the process;
- clarity of vision on a small set of outcome-oriented objectives.

one-sidedness. However, the alternative is potentially neglecting the public health implications of epidemiological research.

When applying epidemiology to public policy in a given country, difficult decisions have to be made about the relevance of research done elsewhere. It is usually impossible – and probably unnecessary – for major studies to be repeated. However, local evidence is often required before local decision-makers accept the arguments for policy change or costly interventions. The local evidence produces a "body count," which can create the impetus for preventive actions.

Framing health policy

In framing health policy, using comparative data on mortality and disability helps to:

- weigh the effects of non-fatal health outcomes on overall population health;
- inform debates on priorities for health service delivery and planning; and research and development of the health sector.[3]

It is easier to both plan and evaluate programmes with a summary measure such as the disability-adjusted life-year (DALY) because it accounts for both mortality and incidence. Changes in either parameter are reflected in a standard way which can be used to track changes over time (Chapter 2).

Almost all policies affect health. Policy decisions by a wide range of agencies – both governmental and nongovernmental – have a significant impact on health. Concern for health and equity is needed in all areas of public policy, as:

- agricultural policies influence the availability, price and quality of meat and dairy products;
- advertising and fiscal policies influence the price and availability of cigarettes or healthy foods such as fruit; and,
- transport policies influence the extent of urban air pollution and the risk of traffic accidents.

This broad social policy approach contrasts with much health policy, which has been directed predominantly towards individuals or groups and has paid little attention to action at the population level.

The Ottawa Charter for Health Promotion (1985) – claims that health is influenced by a wide range of policy decisions.[4] The Charter made it clear that health policy is not simply the responsibility of health departments. The Bangkok Charter for Health Promotion in a Globalized World (2005) states that health promotion depends on empowering all sectors and addressing the global influences on health.[5] (Box 10.2)

One goal of a healthy public policy is health promotion (enabling people to increase control over, and to improve, their own health). Each individual plays a role in achieving the goals of healthy public policy.

Box 10.2. Bangkok Charter for Health Promotion[5]

The Bangkok Charter calls for all sectors and settings to:

- **advocate** for health based on human rights and solidarity;
- **invest** in sustainable policies, actions and infrastructure to address the determinants of health;
- **build capacity** for policy development, leadership, health promotion practice, knowledge transfer and research, and health literacy;
- **regulate and legislate** to ensure a high level of protection from harm and enable equal opportunity for health and well being for all people;
- **build alliances** with public, private, nongovernmental and international organizations and civil society to create sustainable actions.

To do this, four key commitments are identified to make the promotion of health:

- central to the global development agenda
- a core responsibility for all of government
- a key focus of communities and civil society
- a requirement for good corporate practice

Health policy in practice

The time-scale for the application of epidemiological research to policy varies; especially with chronic diseases, it can be measured in decades rather than years. Box 10.3 outlines the findings of research on coronary heart disease and the resulting policy

---

Box 10.3. Evolution of national policy:coronary heart disease

By the early 1950s, the public health significance of coronary heart disease was recognized, although little was known about the risk factors. However, the link between serum cholesterol and coronary heart disease was suspected on the basis of animal experiments, and pathologists had shown that cholesterol was a major component of atherosclerotic lesions in humans. International studies began to explore the role of dietary fat in the 1950s, and major cohort studies began. By the end of the 1950s observational evidence was accumulating on the importance of elevated serum cholesterol, hypertension and smoking as the major risk factors for coronary heart disease.

The observational studies were complemented in the 1960s by the first trials that tested the effect of attempts to alter dietary fat intake on rates of coronary heart disease. Many of these trials were flawed and none produced a convincing effect individually, although the trends were consistent. It was soon recognized that definitive trials of dietary factors and coronary heart disease were impracticable and attention turned to the effect of blood pressure- and cholesterol-lowering drugs.

From a policy perspective, many official pronouncements were made, beginning in 1960 with the first statement of the American Heart Association. In 1985 the National Consensus Development Conference in the USA signalled an increased emphasis on the prevention of coronary heart disease, in particular through attempts to lower cholesterol levels in both high-risk people and the population at large. This programme included a national education campaign on high cholesterol levels, a laboratory standardization programme, and continued efforts to lower cholesterol levels through strategies aimed at both the population and high-risk groups.

In 2003, the Centres for Disease Control and Prevention (CDC) developed a comprehensive national public health action plan for heart health promotion. The aim of this plan was to chart a course by which collaborating public health agencies, all interested partners and the public at large, would promote national goals for preventing heart disease and stroke over the next two decades.

It has taken over 50 years for comprehensive prevention and control policies for coronary heart disease and stroke to be introduced in the United States. However, the emphasis of public policy on coronary heart disease still lies, to a large extent, in attempts to influence individual behaviour, both for members of the health professions and for the public.

decisions in the United States. This examples shows the steps in the evolution of public policy in parallel to the health-care planning process discussed later in this chapter.

In most countries, relatively little attention has been directed towards long-term community-based prevention programmes for heart diseases and even less to facilitating healthy dietary habits, physical activity, and discouraging smoking at the population level. However, coronary heart disease is the first major chronic noncommunicable disease to receive such close attention from both researchers and policy-makers. It is possible that more rapid action will be taken to control other major chronic noncommunicable diseases on the basis of the experience gained, as, for example, with the control of tobacco use. (Box 10.4)

For communicable diseases, action has usually been more swift because infectious epidemics are seen as a more immediate national threat, and a threat to the economy. SARS, which affected only 8000 people causing 1300 deaths, was estimated to cost 30–140 billion USD. Travel and trade were seriously affected by the fear of infection, and costly preventive programs were established in many countries. Resources were rapidly invested in the development of alert and response mechanisms, and the International Health Regulations (see Box 7.2) were revised accordingly. Epidemiologists, working with a wide range of partners, were crucial to the efforts in bringing this epidemic under control.

Box 10.4. Evolution of global policy: The Framework Convention on Tobacco Control

Major global progress has been made with efforts to control tobacco – the most important preventable risk factor for chronic diseases – and provides a good example of the way in which countries can use collective epidemiological knowledge to affect change. The epidemiological evidence for the harmful effects of tobacco ultimately led to the Framework Convention on Tobacco Control in February 2006, the first health treaty adopted by the Member States of WHO. As of the end of 2006, 142 countries – representing 77% of the world's population – had ratified this Convention.

Effective primordial prevention – which means stopping the promotion of cigarettes and preventing people from becoming smokers – requires strong government regulation and fiscal policies for tobacco control.[6] The Framework Convention was developed in response to the globalization of the tobacco epidemic. The tobacco epidemic is exacerbated by a variety of cross-border factors, including trade liberalization, direct foreign investment, global marketing, transnational tobacco advertising, promotion and sponsorship, and the international movement of contraband and counterfeit cigarettes. This Convention represents a major shift by developing a regulatory strategy to address addictive substances. In contrast to previous drug control treaties, the Convention addresses reduction of demand as well as reduction of supply. Successful implementation of the Framework Convention will help to save millions of lives.

Health planning

In this section, we illustrate the process of planning for, and evaluating, a health intervention directed towards a specific disease. The same process should be adopted in broader interventions, such as the development of a national care programme for the elderly, or a new approach to the delivery of primary health care in rural areas.

The systematic use of epidemiological principles and methods for the planning and evaluation of health services is an important aspect of modern epidemiology. From assessing the value of specific treatments it is a short step to assessing the more general performance of health services. The ultimate – though perhaps unrealistic – goal is to develop a transparent process for setting priorities and allocating scarce health care resources.

Because of the limited resources available for health care in all countries, choices have to be made between alternative strategies for improving health (see Chapter 6). In the poorest countries, only a few dollars per person are available for public health services. Consequently, a large proportion of health service costs are met by individuals or their families, so-called "out-of-pocket" expenses. At the other extreme, in the United States of America, approximately 5 600 USD is spent per person on health services each year.

The planning cycle

Fig. 10.1 outlines the stages involved in the health planning process and provides a useful framework for ensuring that the information required by policy-makers is iden-tified. The process is a cycle of the following steps:

- assessing the burden
- identifying the causes
- measuring the effectiveness of existing interventions
- determining efficiency
- implementing interventions
- monitoring activities and measuring progress.

Figure 10.1. The health planning cycle

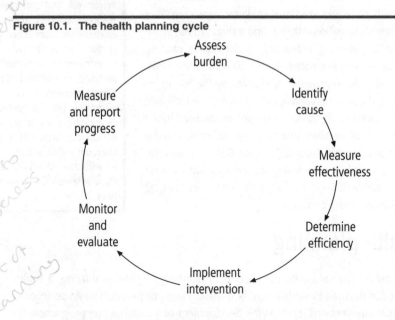

Usually, only part of the information needed for making decisions is available and it always has to be critically assessed. If the information is insufficient, new data have to be collected for appropriate policy choices. To achieve transparency in decision-making, all assumptions should be clearly stated. This can be applied to other health policy issues. Even so, caution is required (Box 10.5).[7]

Epidemiology is involved at all stages of planning. The cyclical nature of the process indicates the importance of monitoring and evaluation to determine whether the interventions have had the desired effects. The process is repetitive because each cycle of intervention usually has only a small impact on the burden of illness, and repeated intervention is required.

A simplified example of the planning cycle is the STEPwise framework for planning (Fig. 10.2). This approach – developed by WHO for health planning in the context of chronic diseases – has relevance to other major policy issues.[8]

Assessing burden

The first step in the planning process is to measure the overall health status of the community. Where no information exists, simple information on the prevalence of major risk factors for disease – especially those few major, but modifiable risk factors which predict chronic diseases – can be collected using the STEPwise approach to Surveillance (STEPS) (Box 10.6) and may be sufficient to initiate a planned response to these diseases.

Mortality and morbidity

Ideally, the process of measuring the burden of disease and injury should include indicators that fully assess the effects of disease on society. Mortality data reflect only one aspect of health and are of limited value for conditions that rarely fatal. Measures of morbidity reflect another important aspect of the burden of illness. The consequences of disease – impairment, disability and handicap

> **Box 10.5. A word of caution: the reality of planning**
>
> Most planning models, including the stepwise framework, assume a rational, sequential approach. While the stepwise framework has the benefits of offering a rational process and rallying multiple disciplines around an acceptable course of action, it does not automatically resolve the difficulties encountered in planning disease prevention and control programmes. The reality is that public health action is incremental, opportunistic, and reversals or changes of direction occur constantly.
>
> The priority accorded to different health programmes is partly a result of the broader political climate. It is important to identify – and ideally predict – the national or sub-national political climate and to capitalize on opportunities to advance health.
>
> The priorities of individual political leaders can be dramatically shaped by private experiences. There are many examples of leaders who, after being personally touched by disease, have subsequently made that disease a national priority for action. These people can be important allies for change.

Figure 10.2. The stepwise framework for prevention[8]

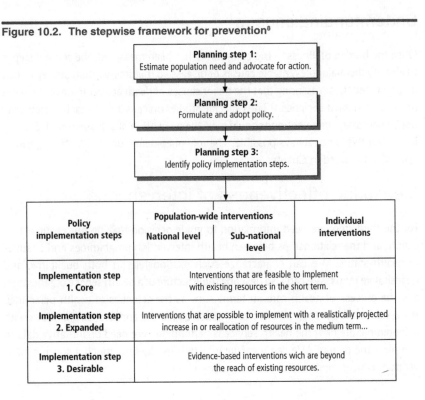

Box 10.6. Estimating burden of risk factors for chronic disease

WHO has developed a tool to help countries assess their risk factor profiles – the STEPwise approach to Surveillance (STEPS).

WHO STEPS focuses on building capacity in low- and middle-income countries to collect small amounts of high-quality risk factor data.

- Step 1 collects information about tobacco use, alcohol consumption, diet and physical activity by questionnaires;
- Step 2 collects data on blood pressure, height and weight by physical measurements;
- Step 3 collects blood samples for measuring lipids and glucose.

Although most countries have the resources for Steps 1 and 2, Step 3 is expensive and not suitable for all settings. STEPS is designed to adapt to local needs, and offer expanded modules (on oral health and stroke, for example) while encouraging collection of standardized data, to facilitate comparisons between and within countries, and over time.

The STEPS Manual can be downloaded from: http://www.who.int/chp/steps

(see Chapter 2) – also need to be measured. The burden – in terms of the number of cases or population level health damage created by a particular factor – is called its public health impact. Health impact assessment has become an important tool in health policy development – initially for environmental health – but now used in all policy areas.

Summary population measures

Summary measures of the burden of disease and injury must be accurate and simple to interpret (see Chapter 2). Many assumptions are involved in the use of these indices and caution is required in their interpretation, but they are intended to make the choice of options in health policy and planning more transparent.[9]

Rapid assessment

Rapid assessment is a defined field of epidemiological research that uses methods to assess health problems and evaluate health programmes in low- and middle-income countries as efficiently as possible. Rapid assessment includes methods for small-area surveys and sampling, surveillance, screening and individual risk assessment, community indicators of risk and health status, and case-control studies for evaluation.[10]

Understanding causes

Once the burden of illness in the community has been measured, the second step is to identify the major preventable causes of disease so that intervention strategies can be developed. It is reassuring that the major causes of death appear to have the same risk factors in most societies.[11] Thus specific studies on causation in each society may not be necessary. Interventions should have the prevention of disease as their primary focus, but this is not always possible. The role of epidemiology in identifying causal factors is discussed in Chapter 5.

Measuring effectiveness of interventions

For the third step, we need information to guide decision-making on resource allocation, and the relationships between health intervention programmes and changes in health status. We can characterize such relationships in both qualitative and quantitative terms. We can also describe the structure of a health service organization and the process of health care, in terms such as the activities of health personnel. However – although they are important – such qualitative approaches provide us with a limited picture how the health service is performing. We need quantitative data to complete the picture. We can measure effectiveness by how much a specific intervention reduces morbidity or mortality (Box 10.7).

Assessing efficiency

Efficiency is a measure of the relationship between the results achieved and resources expended. It provides the basis for the optimal use of resources and covers the relationship between costs and effectiveness of an intervention. This is an area that combines epidemiology and health economics.

There are two main approaches to assessing efficiency.

- *Cost-effectiveness analysis* seeks to determine the costs and effectiveness of an intervention or its alternatives to determine the relative degree to which they result in the desired health outcome. The preferred intervention, or alternative, is one which requires the least cost to produce a given level of effectiveness. In health, cost-effectiveness looks at the ratio of financial expenditure and effectiveness: dollars per life year gained, dollars per case prevented, dollars per quality-adjusted life year gained, and so on (Box 10.8).

- *Cost-benefit analysis* considers the economic costs of a defined type of disease or injury and the costs of prevention. Included in the economic costs of the disease would be the cost of medical care and rehabilitation, the loss of earnings and the estimated social cost of a death. "Willingness-to-pay" can be used to determine what the social cost of a death is: for high-income countries, this analysis usually produces a value of life at a few million US dollars. In cost-benefit analyses, both the numerator and denominator are expressed in monetary terms. The benefit of an intervention is the avoided cost of the disease cases, and the cost of the intervention is the direct cost of implementing preventive actions. If the cost-benefit analysis shows that economic benefits of the intervention (or the benefit of preventing an additional case) are greater than the costs of prevention, the intervention would be economically profitable. Interventions that cost more than the calculated economic benefit may still be considered attractive due to the improved population health status that they achieve.

> **Box 10.7. Factors determining effectiveness of interventions**
>
> The effectiveness of interventions in the community is determined by many factors.
>
> - How well the intervention works in the research setting: if the intervention does not work under ideal conditions, it is unlikely to work in the community. Close attention to diagnosis, long-term management and follow-up, often happens only in randomized controlled trials. Such trials have shown, for example, that the treatment of mild hypertension reduces rates of fatal and nonfatal stroke by about 40%. However – due to problems with compliance and patient selection – antihypertensive treatment is less effective in the community.
> - The ability to screen for, and diagnose the disease affects outcome (see Chapter 6).
> - The intervention should be used by all who could benefit; this means that it is available, affordable, and acceptable to the community.

> **Box 10.8. Oral rehydration therapy - good value for money**
>
> Cost-effectiveness also helps identify neglected opportunities by highlighting interventions that are relatively inexpensive, yet have the potential to reduce the disease burden. An good example is oral rehydration therapy. Oral rehydration therapy is given at home, bypassing health services and thus increasing its cost-effectiveness. Although it does not reduce the incidence of diarrhoea, oral rehydration therapy reduces its severity and associated deaths. At 2–4 USD per life-year saved, this is seen as good value and good public policy. Oral rehydration therapy has been widely adopted, saving millions of lives.[9]

Cost-effectiveness analysis is easier to perform than cost-benefit analysis, since the measure of effectiveness does not need to be given a monetary value. Table 10.1 summarizes the estimated costs for each extra disability-adjusted life year gained as a result of various procedures for preventing chronic diseases. These figures assume a constant cost of implementation.

Table 10.1. Preventing and treating chronic noncommunicable disease: the amount of health 1 million USD will buy.[9]

Service or intervention	Cost per DALY (USD)	DALYs averted per 1 million USD
Tax on tobacco products	3–50	20 000–330 000
Treatment of myocardial infarction with inexpensive drugs	10–25	40 000–100 000
Treatment of myocardial infarction with inexpensive drugs plus streptokinase	600–750	1 300–1 600
Lifelong treatment of cardiovascular disease with a daily "polypill"	700–1 000	1 000–1 400
Surgery for specific high-risk cases	25 000+	Less than 40
Surgery for less severe coronary artery disease	Very high	Very few

Although these estimates are based on approximate information and many assumptions, they are useful to policy-makers who have to set priorities. The measurement of efficiency requires many assumptions and it should be used very cautiously; it is not value-free and can serve only as a general guideline. The best evidence for cost-effectiveness studies comes from randomized controlled trials or systematic reviews and the weakest evidence comes from small case series or surveys of expert opinion.

Three examples of cost-benefit analysis for environmental pollution are given in Table 9.2. Health planners in all countries are interested in determining the economic aspects of proposed health programs. In low- and middle-income countries this interest has been sparked by the Millennium Development Goals (see Chapter 7), but also results from the recognition of equity as a key objective of health policy. Cost-effectiveness studies have become more widely disseminated – and easier to do – with the tools and regional databases provided by WHO-CHOICE (Box 10.9) and the Disease Control Priorities Project.[9]

Box 10.9. Choosing interventions that are cost-effective: WHO-CHOICE

WHO-CHOICE assembles regional databases on the costs, population health impacts, and cost-effectiveness of key health interventions. It also provides a tool for adapting regional results to countries. WHO-CHOICE provides analysts with a method for assessing the efficiency – in a particular setting – of current and proposed interventions.[12]

Implementing interventions

The fifth step in the planning process involves setting targets, and making sure that they can be reached. We need to anticipate, and address, the problems that are likely to arise as a result of the decisions that have been made. For example, if we plan to use mammography to screen for breast cancer, we need to ensure that the necessary equipment and personnel are available. We also need to set specific quantified targets, such as "to reduce the incidence of advanced breast cancer from 30% to 20% over a five-year period." This type of target-setting is essential if we want to formally assess the success of an intervention. Of course, in practice, it is hard to isolate the impact of the specific intervention from other changes in society.

Monitoring activities and measuring progress

The final step in the planning process is monitoring and measuring progress. Monitoring is the continuous follow-up of activities to ensure that they are proceeding according to plan. We need to tailor monitoring to specific programs, the success of which we can measure with short-term, intermediate, and long-term criteria. Table 10.2 provides a specific example of all the planning steps.

Table 10.2. Health planning: the case of raised blood pressure

Burden	Population surveys of blood pressure and control of hypertension
Causation	Ecological studies (salt and blood pressure)
	Observational studies (weight and blood pressure)
	Experimental studies (weight reduction)
Effectiveness	Randomized controlled trials
	Evaluation of screening programmes
	Studies of compliance
Efficiency	Cost-effectiveness studies
Implementation	National control programmes for high blood pressure, ideally based on absolute risk
Monitoring and measuring progress	Assessment of personnel and equipment Effect on quality of life Repeated population surveys of blood pressure

In this case – for a community blood pressure program – monitoring and evaluation could include regular assessment of:

- personnel training;
- the availability and accuracy of blood pressure measuring devices (structural);
- the appropriateness of case-finding and management procedures (process evaluation);
- the effect on blood pressure levels in treated patients (outcome evaluation).

To measure progress, we may need to repeat burden-of-illness measurements in the population. Trends in population levels of risk factors and the uptake of interventions are often used to estimate the impact of various interventions

The full value of epidemiological research is realized only when its results are translated into health policy and programmes. Translating evidence into policy remains a major challenge for epidemiologists, but the field makes crucial contributions to health planning and evaluation.

Study questions

10.1 Apply the principles of the Bangkok Charter for Health Promotion to the development of healthy public policy regarding the prevention of tobacco use in children.

10.2 Outline the steps of the health planning cycle with reference to the problem of falls in the elderly.

10.3 How could the parameters described in Table 10.2 be used to influence health policy and planning in your country?

References

1. *World health report 2000: Health systems: improving performance.* Geneva, World Health Organization, 2000.

2. *Prevention of chronic diseases: a vital investment.* Geneva, World Health Organization, 2005.

3. Van Der Maas PJ. Applications of Summary Measures of Population Health. In: Ezzati M et al., eds. *Summary Measures of Population Health. Concepts, ethics, measurement and applications.* Geneva, World Health Organization, 2002:53-60.

4. *Ottowa charter for health promotion,* 1986. http://www.who.int/hpr/NPH/docs/ottawa_charter_hp.pdf.

5. Bangkok charter for health promotion in a globalized world, 2005. http://www.who.int/healthpromotion/conferences/6gchp/bangkok_chart er/en/

6. WHO framework convention on tobacco control. Geneva, World Health Organization, 2003.

7. Tugwell P, Bennett KJ, Sackett DL, Haynes RB. The measurement iterative loop: a framework for the critical appraisal of need, benefits and costs of health interventions. *J Chronic Dis* 1985;38:339-51.

8. Bonita R, Douglas K, Winkelmann R, De Courten M. The WHO STEPwise approach to surveillance (STEPS) of noncommunicable disease risk factors. In: McQueen DV, Puska P, eds. *Global Risk Factor Surveillance.* London, Kluwer Academic/Plenum Publishers, 2003:9-22.

9. Jamison DT, Breamn JG, Measham AR, Alleyne G, Claeson M, Evans DB, et al., editors. *Disease control priorities in developing countries.* New York, Oxford University Press, 2006.

10. Smith GS. Development of rapid epidemiologic assessment methods to evaluate health status and delivery of health services. *Int J Epidemiol* 1989;18:S2-15.

11. Yusuf S, Hawken S, Ounpuu S, Dans T, Avezum A, Lanas F, et al. Effect of potentially modifiable risk factors associated with myocardial infarction in 52 countries (the INTERHEART study): case-control study. *Lancet* 2004;364:937-952.

12. Baltussen R, Adam T, Tan Torres T, Hutubessy R, Acharya A, Evans DB, et al. Generalized cost-effectiveness analysis: a guide. In: Jones AM, ed. *The Elgar Companion To Health Economics,* Edward Elgar Press; 2006: 479-491.

Chapter 11
First steps in practical epidemiology

Key messages

- An interesting career in epidemiology depends on a willingness to learn more about diseases and risk factors.
- Knowing how to select reading material – and how to appraise its relevance and validity – is an important part of keeping informed about new developments.
- Doing epidemiological research well depends on coming up with good questions, writing clear protocols, obtaining ethical approval, and publishing and applying the results.
- This work is made easier by the many online resources that are freely available, including databases, analytical tools, references, and teaching guidelines.

Introduction

If this book has been successful, you should be keen to apply what you have learnt to practical work in epidemiology. To do this, you should keep an open mind, and be always on the lookout for good research questions. You need to think about how to apply the right study design to answer your question (Chapter 3), how to get approval and funding, how to make sure that it hasn't already been done, how to do the research well, and how to write up, present, and publish your findings.

Specific diseases

One place to start is continually learning more about specific diseases or public health problems. A basic understanding of disease epidemiology requires knowledge of the items listed in Table 11.1. Rare, emerging, or rapidly evolving diseases are often the subject of ongoing research to establish these very characteristics.

You should seek to complement your epidemiological knowledge with what is known about the pathology, clinical treatment, pharmacology, rehabilitation and economic impact of a disease. More detailed knowledge of engineering or sanitation aspects of prevention, economic impact or changing patterns may be needed for particular areas of public health practice.

Rather than focus on a specific disease, you may choose to focus on a specific risk factor such as tobacco smoking or pesticide exposure. This would also involve studying the literature and doing research on the particular risk its route of exposure to humans, and the mechanisms by which it affects health (Table 11.2).

Table 11.1. Basic epidemiological information about a disease

Natural history in the individual:
- development with age (cohort basis)
- early indicators (for screening)
- impact of different treatments
- possibility of cure
- need for care
- social impact

Etiology:
- specific causal factors
- other risk factors

Development in the community:
- time trends
- variations with age (cross-sectional basis)

Differences in occurrence:
- sex
- ethnic group
- social class
- occupation
- geographical area

Possibilities for prevention:
- specific actions to address causal factors and underlying determinants
- general actions to address other risk factors
- impact of medical services including screening and early detection
- impact of health policy

Critical reading

Keeping informed, even in a narrow field, is difficult because of the huge quantity of material that is published. Finding, sorting through, and understanding relevant and valid information is a crucial skill that can only be acquired through a lot of practice. However, the effort spent learning to appraise papers is repaid when it comes to designing research, as the same questions apply.

One approach is to first categorize papers into four broad types – most epidemiological research papers are either on the natural history of disease; its geographic distribution; its causes; treatment; or diagnostic tests. The level of evidence that any particular study will be able to provide is linked to its design. In general, levels of evidence are considered to progress from expert opinion, through case-series, to cohort studies, randomized controlled trials and systematic reviews, but it is important to consider the quality and validity of any one example in addition to its relative position on the ladder.

When reading a paper, you may wish to consider the following questions, in this order.

Table 11.2. Basic epidemiological information about a hazard

Driving forces	Examples
policy	tobacco advertising legislation
economics	tobacco tax, cigarette pricing
technological developments	catalytic converters that reduce air pollution
Sources of the hazard	
specific processes	coal burning and air pollution
impact of other factors	meteorological factors and air pollution
daily or seasonal variations	ozone levels
Historical and geographic trends	
Factors influencing the level of human exposure	**Health effects**
age, sex, ethnic group differences	mechanism of causation
diet, physical activity, climate factors	early biochemical or physiological indicators of damage
work activities	means to prevent exposure and health effects
other behavioural factors	

What is the research question?

- The first step is to determine the objectives of the study – the question that the authors wish to address or the hypothesis that they wish to test.

If valid, are the results relevant to my work?

- If yes, keep reading.
- If no, start again with another paper.

What kind of study is this?

- Cross-sectional studies address questions about the prevalence of a disease or risk factor.
- Cohort studies address questions about natural history or prognosis and causation.
- Case-control or cohort studies identify possible causal factors.
- Randomized controlled trials are usually the most appropriate design for answering questions about the efficacy of treatment or other interventions.

What is the study population?

- Who is included and who is excluded?
- Are the subjects a sample of the target population?
- If not, why not?
- How have the samples been selected?
- Is there evidence of random selection, as opposed to systematic, or self-selection?
- What possible sources of bias are there in the selection strategy?
- Is the sample large enough to answer the question being addressed?

For experimental studies, are the methods well described?

- How were the subjects assigned to treatment or intervention: randomly or by some other method?
- What control groups were included (placebo, untreated controls, both or neither?
- How were the treatments compared?
- Were measurements supported by quality assurance procedures?
- Is the hypothesis clearly stated in statistical terms?
- Is the statistical analysis appropriate, and is it presented in sufficient detail?
- If this is a randomized controlled trial, was the study done with an "intention-to-treat" analysis - e.g. are all the people who entered the study accounted for?
- Were the outcome or effects measured objectively?

For observational studies, are the methods well described?

- Was the data collection process adequate (including questionnaire design and pre-testing)?
- What techniques were used to handle non-response and/or incomplete data?
- If a cohort study, was the follow-up rate sufficiently high?
- If a case-control study, are the controls appropriate, and adequately matched?

How are the data presented?

- Are there sufficient graphs and/or tables?
- Are the numbers consistent? Is the entire sample accounted for?
- Are standard deviations presented with means, confidence intervals, or other statistics, as well as the raw data?

Evaluating and interpreting the results

If you have been persuaded so far that the study is valid and relevant, it is worth proceeding.

If it is an experimental study,

- Do the authors find a difference between the treatment and control groups?
- If there is no difference, and you can rule out the possibility of a Type II error (see Chapter 4), then this is a negative study – which does not mean that the results are of no consequence.
- If the authors have found a difference, are you confident that it is not due to chance (a Type I error, see Chapter 4), or bias?
- If there is a statistically significant difference, is it enough of a difference to be clinically significant?

If it is an observational study

- Were the findings in the control group consistent with what you would expect – are the averages similar to the general population?
- Do the authors find a difference between exposed and control groups or cases and controls?
- Can Type I or Type II errors be ruled out?

- Is there a statistically significant difference between groups?
- Could the results be of public health significance, even though the difference is not statistically significant? (This may highlight the need for a larger study.)

Final evaluation
In weighing the evidence, you should ask the following questions

- Was the research question worth asking in the first place, and what could be the consequences of the various possible answers?
- Did the research provide suggestions for action?
- Has the author made an adequate attempt to answer the question?
- Could the study design have been improved?
- Does missing information prevent you from fully evaluating the study?
- Did the author account for results of previous studies?

If you are satisfied that the article provides you with valid and relevant information, then it is logical to use this information in your work, while keeping alert to any further developments.

Planning a research project

Students in many basic epidemiology courses are given the task of designing a study. In some situations students are expected to do the study and analyse the data. There is a natural progression from critical reading to the design of studies. The same questions apply, and the same approach (as outlined above) can be used. Designing a study with help from an experienced tutor is a good way of learning the principles and methods of epidemiology.

The steps involved in planning a research project include:

- choosing the project
- writing the protocol
- getting approval
- doing the research
- analysing the data
- disseminating the results.

Choosing a project

Your supervisors should take an active role in selecting the topic and contacting any participants in the community. Students' projects should not be too ambitious because of the inevitable shortage of time and resources. Ideally, they should be of local significance and of relevance to some health service agency, a member of which could act as a co-supervisor.

Student projects may focus on a wide range of subjects, for example:

- environmental contamination and potential health risks around a waste incinerator;
- attitudes and behaviour in relation to the wearing of crash helmets;
- use of mosquito nets;

- storage of pesticides;
- uptake of antenatal care by first-time mothers.

Writing the protocol

Once you have established – through an extensive literature search – that your proposed research has not already been done, or is worth repeating, you need to write the research protocol. You should consult the relevant consensus guidelines for the type of study that you want to do, to make sure that you cover all the points (Table 11.3). In general, a protocol should explain:

- What you intend to do: a clear description of the problem and your approach to solving it.
- A justification of the importance of the research question, and how it will contribute to knowledge.
- A description of the population, setting, intervention or observation.
- Details of the study design which should include:

  - the sampling strategy,
  - numbers of participants,
  - variables of interest, including potential confounding variables,
  - data collection methods, including pre-testing,
  - quality assurance,
  - data recording and data management
  - data processing and analysis.

- Budget and timetable (include funding sources and all resources needed).
- Roles and responsibilities of all involved.
- The ethical review committee to whom the proposal will be submitted for approval.
- Publication plan: how you will disseminate and apply the results.
- Plans for any community feedback.

Table 11.3. Consensus guidelines on research design and reporting

Subject area	Guidelines	Web address
authorship	Vancouver guidelines (International Committee of Medical Journal Editors)	http://www.icmje.org/index.html
general publication ethics	COPE	http://www.publicationethics.org.uk
meta-analysis of observational studies	MOOSE	http://www.consort-statement.org/ news.html#moose
non-randomized tests of interventions	TREND	http://www.ajph.org/chi/content/full /94/3/361
randomized controlled trials	CONSORT	http://www.consort-statement.org
research ethics	Declaration of Helsinki	http://www.wma.net/e/policy/b3.htm
studies of diagnostic accuracy	STARD	http://www.consort-statement.org/ stardstatement.htm
systematic reviews and meta-analyses of randomized controlled trials	QUOROM	http://www.consort-statement.org/ evidence.html#quorom

Research protocols are subject to intense scrutiny, and are the basis on which you are going to seek funding and ethics approval for your study. Some journals solicit protocols for peer review, in the same way as research papers. Practices vary, but if your protocol survives peer review and is published by the journal, the editors will often undertake to review the paper that contains the main results of the study.

Doing the research

Once you have written the protocol, it needs to be circulated for comments and revised as necessary. With major epidemiological studies there is often a long delay between preparing the protocol and starting the project, caused by the processing of a grant application. Students' projects should be designed so that they can be done quickly, as the time available is often very limited.

Students' projects should not require major resources, and the supervisor should be responsible for acquiring any that are necessary. The supervisor should also be charged with submitting the project for ethical approval in good time.

Group projects require a reasonable division of labour and it is often helpful if one member of the group communicates with the supervisor. You need to review your progress together regularly, and allow time to pretest questionnaires and do a pilot study of the sampling and data collection process.

Your project should end with a verbal presentation to the whole class (preceded, if possible, by a rehearsal) followed by a written report, which could be circulated to interested people. The report could be used for teaching purposes or as a basis for further studies.

Analysing the data

There is a wide choice of software for statistics and epidemiology, ranging from spreadsheets which can do limited analyses, through software made for specific analyses, to "all-purpose" software which can do almost all the statistical analyses required for epidemiological research. A catalogue of epidemiological resources which are available free or at minimal cost has been produced by Epidemiology Monitor (http://www.epimonitor.net). Rothman's Episheet program can be downloaded from http://77www.oup-usa.org/epi/rothman. Public domain programs, such as "OpenEpi" or the CDC's 'Epi Info'™ are also distributed free; commercial programs can cost as much as several thousand US dollars.

In choosing software, you may wish to evaluate how the program handles data entry and missing variables, what the program's capacity is for updating and merging data sets, the types of analysis that it can do, and the presence of any report-writing features or graphics and mapping options.

Getting published

You should think about where you are going to submit your work for publication throughout the planning stages. The best way to resolve disputes over authorship is to avoid them in the first place, which means deciding early who in your research group is going to be an author – and how much of the writing each of you will do.

Guidelines for journal submission often contain very useful information about design and reporting specifications, and many of these are impossible to correct in retrospect. You should consult the relevant consensus guidelines (see Table 11.3) for the type of study you are doing, and make sure that your protocol covers all the points. Your funding source may stipulate that you have to publish in an open access journal, and you will need to register an experimental study with an approved registry to fulfill minimum requirements for publication with major journals.

Further reading

There is no shortage of reading material in epidemiology. Table 11.4 contains a list of relevant peer-reviewed journals. Much epidemiological research is published in general medical journals, and some of these journals have a policy of making such research freely available on the web when it is relevant to developing countries. All the content of open access journals are free to readers and WHO runs a collaboration with major publishers to make all the content of their journals free or low-priced to institutions in developing countries. This is called the HINARI initiative (Box 11.1).

Table 11.5 has recommendations for some advanced textbooks. Nongovernmental, intergovernmental and

---

Box 11.1. The Health InterNetwork Access to Research Initiative (HINARI)

The Health InterNetwork Access to Research Initiative (HINARI) provides free or very low-cost online access to the major journals in biomedical and related social sciences to local, not-for-profit institutions in developing countries. Established in January 2002, more than 70 publishers offer their content to HINARI. Participating institutions need computers connected to the Internet with a high-speed link. Details on how to apply for registration can be found on the WHO web site (http://www.who.int/hinari/en).

Table 11.4. Examples of peer-reviewed journals that publish epidemiological research

American Journal of Epidemiology	http://aje.oxfordjournals.org/
American Journal of Public Health	http://www.ajph.org/
Annals of Epidemiology	http://www.annalsofepidemiology.org/
Bulletin of the World Health Organization	http://www.who.int/bulletin/en/
Cadernos de Saúde Pública	http://www.ensp.fiocruz.br/csp/
Emerging Infectious Diseases	http://www.cdc.gov/ncidod/EID/
Environmental Health Perspectives	
Environmental Research	
Epidemiologia e prevenzione	http://www.zadig.it/eprev/
Epidemiological Reviews	http://epirev.oxfordjournals.org/
Epidemiology	http://www.epidem.com/
European Journal of Epidemiology	http://www.springerlink.com/link.asp?id = 102883
International Journal of Epidemiology	
Journal of Clinical Epidemiology	http://journals.elsevierhealth.com/periodicals/jce
Journal of Epidemiology and Community Health	http://jech.bmjjournals.com/
Public Library of Science Medicine	http://medicine.plosjournals.org
Revista de Saúde Pública	http://www.fsp.usp.br/rsp/
Revista Panamerican de Salud Publica	http://revista.paho.org/
Revue d'épidémiologie et de santé publique	
The British Medical Journal	http://bmj.bmjjournals.com/
The Lancet	http://www.thelancet.com/
Weekly Epidemiological Record	http://www.who.int/wer/en/

governmental agencies also publish vast quantities of useful epidemiological information, and these sources should be systematically consulted for background reading
on a particular topic.

Table 11.5. Suggestions for further reading in epidemiology

Baker D, Kjellstrom T, Calderon R, Pasides H, eds. *Environmental epidemiology.* Document WHO/SDE/OEH/99.7, Geneva, World Health Organization, 1999. (order from: SMI Books, Stevenage, United Kingdom, webmaster @ earthprint.com)

Bradford Hill A. *Principles of Medical Statistics,* 12th ed. Lubrecht & Cramer Ltd, 1991

Checkoway H, Pearce N, Crawford-Brown D. Research methods in occupational epidemiology. New York, Oxford University Press, 1989.

Coggon D, Rose G, Barker DJP. *Epidemiology for the uninitiated.* London, BMJ Publishing Group,1997. http://bmj.bmjjournals.com/collections/epidem/epid.shtml

Detels R, McEwen J, Beaglehole R, Tanaka H. *Oxford Textbook of Public Health.* New York, Oxford University Press, 2002. (ISBN: 0 192 630 415)

Friss RH, Sellers TA. *Epidemiology for public health practice.* Maryland, Aspen, 1996.

Gordis, Leon. *Epidemiology*, 2nd ed. Philadelphia, Saunders, 2000.

Halperin W, Baker EL Jr., Monson RR. *Public health surveillance.* New York,Van Nostrand Reinhold, 1992.

Kahn HA. *Statistical methods in epidemiology.* New York, Oxford University Press, 1989.

Kleinbaum DG, Barker N, Sullivan KM. *ActivEpi Companion Textbook*, Springer, 2005. (ISBN: 0 387 955 747)

Lilienfeld DE, Stolley PD. *Foundations of epidemiology*, 3rd ed. New York, Oxford University Press, 1994.

MacMahon B, Trichopolous D. *Epidemiology: Principles & Methods*, 2nd ed. Boston, Little, Brown, 1996. (ISBN 0 316 542 229)

MacMahon B. *Epidemiology: principles and methods.* 2nd ed. Hagerstown, Lippincott-Raven, 1997.

Mausner JS, Kramer S. *Mausner & Bahn Epidemiology: an introductory text.* Philadelphia,W.B. Saunders, 1985.

Meinert, CL. *Clinical trials: design, conduct, and analysis.* New York, Oxford University Press, 1986.

Morton RF, Hebel JR, McCarter RJ. *A study guide to epidemiology and biostatistics.* Jones and Bartlett Publishers; 2004. (ISBN: 0 763 728 756)

Norell SE *A short course in epidemiology.* New York, Raven Press, 1992. (ISBN 0–881678422)

Pearce N. *A short introduction to epidemiology* Occasional Report Series 2. Wellington, Centre for Public Health Research. (ISBN: 0 473 095 602)

Petitti, Diana B. *Meta-analysis, decision analysis, & cost-effectiveness analysis: methods for quantitative synthesis*, 2nd ed. Oxford University Press, 2000. (ISBN: 0 195 133 641)

Rothman KJ, Greenland S. *Modern Epidemiology* Lippincott Williams & Wilkins; 1998 (ISBN: 0 316 757 802)

Rothman KJ. *Epidemiology: An Introduction.* New York, Oxford University Press, 2002. (ISBN: 0 195 135 547)

Sackett DL, Haynes RB, Tugwell P. *Clinical epidemiology: a basic science for clinical medicine.* New York, Little, Brown, 1985.

Szklo M, Nieto FJ. *Epidemiology: beyond the basics.* Gaithersburg, Aspen, 2000. (ISBN: 0 834 206 188)

Wassertheil-Smoller S. *Biostatistics and Epidemiology: A Primer for Health and Biomedical Professionals* Springer, 2004. (ISBN: 0 387 402 926)

Further training

There are many courses that provide postgraduate training in epidemiology (see
Table 11.6 for useful links). Short summer courses, such as the 3-week "Epidemiology
in Action" course offered by the Public Health Agency of Canada, are common in
North America. The European Programme for Intervention Epidemiology Training
(EPIET) is a good source of similar courses in Europe, and the Network of Training
Programs in Epidemiology and Public Health Interventions (TEPHINET) provides
courses in 32 countries. Graduate courses in epidemiology, usually forming part

of a master's programme in public health, are offered by universities worldwide. The Epidemiology Supercourse is a free public library of epidemiology lectures – with contributions from 151 countries and translations in eight languages.

Table 11.6. Useful links to epidemiological software and courses

Annual Summer Programme in Epidemiology and Biostatistics, McGill University	http://www.mcgill.ca/epi-biostat/
Annual Summer Session for Public Health Studies, Harvard University	http://www.hsph.harvard.edu/summer/brochure/
Annual Summer Session in Epidemiology, The University of Michigan	http://www.sph.umich.edu/epid/GSS/
Canadian Field Epidemiology Program	http://www.phac-aspc.gc.ca/cfep-pcet/summer_c_e.html
Chinese Education and Reseach Network	http://www.cernet.edu.cn/
Course material for Epiinfo	http://www.epiinformatics.com/Resources.htm
Critical Appraisal Skills Programme	http://www.phru.nhs.uk/casp/casp.htm
Free Epidata software	http://www.epidata.dk
Free public health software	http://www.brixtonhealth.com/
Interactive Statistical Pages Project	http://statpages.org/
Karolinska Institutet	http://www.bioepi.org/
Open source software	http://www.openepi.com/Menu/OpenEpiMenu.htm
Public domain Epiinfo software	http://www.cdc.gov/Epiinfo/
Summer Program in Intermediate Epidemiology and Biostatistics, PAHO	http://www.paho.org/english/sha/shaforrec.htm
Textbook and CD demo	http://www.activepi.com/
The Epidemiology Supercourse	http://www.pitt.edu/~super1
The Erasmus Summer Programme, Erasmus University Rotterdam	http://www.erasmussummerprogramme.nl/
The European Programme for Intervention Epidemiology Training	http://www.epiet.org/
The Johns Hopkins Graduate Summer Program in Epidemiology	http://www.jhsph.edu/summerEpi
The Network of Training Programs in Epidemiology and Public Health Interventions	http://tephinet.org/
Umeå International School of Public Health	http://www.umu.se/phmed/epidemi/utbildning/index.html
University of Alabama Masters in Public Health – Biostatistics Course	http://statcourse.dopm.uab.edu/

Study questions

11.1 The following is based on the preliminary report of a study designed to assess the value of aspirin in the prevention of coronary heart disease. (The physicians' health study: aspirin for the primary prevention of myocardial infarction. *N Engl J Med* 1988 Apr 7;318:924-6.).

The Physicians' Health Study is a randomized double-blind, placebo-controlled trial testing whether 325mg of aspirin taken every other day reduces mortality from cardiovascular disease. The potentially eligible participants in the study were all male physicians 40 to 84 years of age residing in the United States at the beginning of the study in 1982. Letters of invitation, informed-consent forms, and baseline questionnaires were mailed to 261248 such physicians identified from information on a computer tape obtained from the American Medical Association. By 31 December 1983, 112528 had responded, of whom 59285 were willing to participate in the trial. A large number were excluded during the enrolment phase because of poor compliance (judged by pill counts); physicians with a history of gastric bleeding and intolerance to aspirin were also excluded. 11037 physicians were assigned at random to receive active aspirin and 11034 to receive aspirin placebo.

This study found that aspirin had a strong protective effect against non-fatal myocardial infarction. Would you be happy to prescribe aspirin for the prevention of coronary heart disease?

11.2 The following extract is taken from a paper on asthma mortality in New Zealand, published in the *Lancet* (Wilson JD, Sutherland DC, Thomas AC. Has the change to beta-agonists combined with oral theophylline increased cases of fatal asthma? *Lancet* 1981;1:1235-37.)

Abstract

An apparent increase in young people dying suddenly from acute asthma has been noted in the past 2 years in Auckland. 22 fatal cases were reviewed. Prescribing habits for asthma therapy have been changing in New Zealand, with a considerable increase in the use of oral theophylline drugs, particularly sustained-release preparations, which in many patients have replaced inhaled steroids and cromoglycate. It is suggested that there may be an additive toxicity between theophylline and inhaled B_2-agonists at high doses which produces cardiac arrest.

Methods

Details of deaths from asthma were obtained from the coroner's pathologist, the Auckland Asthma Society, general practitioners, and from the intensive and critical care wards of Auckland Hospital. The doctors and relatives of the patients were contacted and descriptions of mode of death and the pattern of drug administration were obtained. Statistical information on fatal asthma cases in New Zealand in the years 1974–78 was obtained from the New Zealand Department of Health. Necropsies had been performed on the 8 patients referred to the coroner.

Taking into consideration the methods used, would you agree with the suggestion that a toxic drug interaction was leading to an increased risk of death?

Chapter 1

1.1   The fact that there were over 40 times more cholera cases in one district than in the other does not reflect the risk of catching cholera in the two districts. It is not appropriate to compare the number of deaths in the two groups since the population supplied by the Southwark Company was over eight times larger than the population supplied by the Lambeth Company. Death rates (number of deaths divided by the population supplied) must be compared. In fact the death rate in the population supplied by the Southwark Company was over five times greater than that in the Lambeth district.

1.2   The best evidence would come from intervention studies. The 1854 epidemic was controlled in a most dramatic manner when the handle of a water pump was removed. The epidemic died away rapidly, although the evidence suggests (and Snow knew) that the epidemic was already waning before this act. More convincing was the reduction in cholera rates in the population supplied by the Lambeth Company in the period 1849–54 (before the epidemic) after the Company had begun extracting water from a less contaminated part of the River Thames.

1.3   Doctors make a good study group because they comprise a well-defined occupational group with similar socioeconomic status, and are relatively easy to follow up. They are also likely to be interested in health matters and co-operative in this type of study.

1.4   It can be concluded that lung cancer death rates increase dramatically with the number of cigarettes smoked. From the data alone it is not possible to conclude that smoking causes lung cancer; some other factor associated with smoking might be causing the disease. However, in 1964, on the basis of this study and many others, the United States Surgeon General concluded that lung cancer was caused by cigarette smoking.

1.5   The distribution of the population is the first factor to consider. The concentration of cases in one area is interesting only if the population is spread throughout that area. Secondly, it needs to be known whether the search for cases has been as intensive in the areas without cases as in the area with cases. During the Minamata disease outbreak, an intensive search was made throughout the whole region and it was found that several large population centres had no cases.

1.6   The reported occurrence of rheumatic fever has declined dramatically in Denmark since the early 1900s. It could be a real decline although it would be important to try to rule out the influence of changes in diagnostic fashion and reporting practices. Since effective medical treatment for rheumatic fever became available only in the 1940s, most of the decline has been due to socioeconomic improvements, e.g. in housing and nutrition. It is also possible that the responsible organism has become less virulent.

1.7   Men who do not smoke and are not exposed to asbestos dust have the lowest lung cancer rates, followed in increasing order by men exposed to asbestos dust alone, men who smoke but are not exposed to asbestos dust, and finally men who both smoke and are exposed to asbestos dust. This is an example of interaction in which two factors work together to produce a very high rate of disease. From a public health perspective it is important to ensure that people exposed to asbestos dust do not smoke, and, of course, to reduce exposure to the dust.

Chapter 2

2.1 The three measures are prevalence, incidence and cumulative incidence. Prevalence is the proportion of the population affected by a disease or condition at a given point in time and is approximately equal to the incidence multiplied by the duration of disease. Incidence measures the rate at which new events occur in a population; it can take into account variable time periods during which individuals are disease-free. Cumulative incidence measures the denominator (i.e. the population at risk) at only one point in time (usually at the beginning of a study) and thus measures the risk of individuals contracting a disease during a specified period.

2.2 Prevalence is a useful measure of the frequency of non-insulin-dependent diabetes because diabetes has a relatively low incidence and because a very large population and a long study period would be required in order to find sufficient new cases to measure incidence. The variation shown in Table 2.2 could reflect differences in measurement. The adequacy of the methods used in the various surveys would need to be assessed; survey response rates and laboratory methods would have to be looked at, among other things. It should be noted, however, that standard criteria are being applied on the basis of blood glucose levels after a standard glucose load. It is likely that much of the variation in diabetes prevalence is real and due, at least in part, to variations in diet, exercise and other elements of lifestyle.

2.3 The population attributable risk or attributable fraction (population) is calculated as:

$$\frac{30.2-17.7}{30.2} = 0.414$$

corresponding to 41.4%.

2.4 Risk difference and risk ratio.

2.5 Although the relative risk is only about 1.5, the population attributable risk is about 20% (i.e. about 20% of the cases of lung cancer in a typical population of a developed country can be attributed to passive smoking). This is because up to half the population is exposed to passive smoking.

2.6 Age standardization ensures that differences in death rates are not due simply to differences in age distribution in the populations. Standardizing crude rates takes the age distribution out of the picture and therefore allows a comparison of populations with different age structures by using a population with a standard age distribution

2.7 Either rate can be used and even the number of cancer deaths. It all depends on how the information will be interpreted. The number of cases tells you which part of the country would have the largest number of cancer cases needing treatment. The crude rate tells you where the number of case per capita is the highest, but a high crude rate may just indicate that there are many elderly people in that area. However, the age standardized rates tells us where the risk of cancer is highest, which would be the first step in designing epidemiological studies to identify preventable risk factors.

2.8 They reflect the fact that the average life expectancy in Cote d'Ivoire is low and there are not many people in the older age groups (and cancer risk increases with age).

2.9   Without having the age standardized rates for both countries, comparisons
      are not possible. The higher crude rates in Japan could have occurred because
      it has the highest life expectancy in the world and many more older people
      than in Cote d'Ivoire - ie they have populations with radically different age
      distributions.

      In fact, Japan has a an age standardized cancer rate of 119.2 per 100,000
      compared with Cote d'Ivoire (which has a rate of 160.2 per 100,000 - see
      above). With age standardization, Cote d'Ivoire's rate increases and Japanese
      rates decrease.

Chapter 3

3.1 The main epidemiological study designs are the cross-sectional survey, the case-control study, the cohort study and the randomized controlled trial. Their relative strengths and weaknesses are summarized in the text and in Tables 3.3 and 3.4.

3.2 The case-control study would start with cases of bowel cancer, preferably newly diagnosed ones, and a group of controls (without the disease) from the same source population (to avoid selection bias). The cases and controls would be asked about their usual diet in the past. Measurement bias could be a problem. It is difficult to remember past diet with great accuracy, and the development of the disease might influence recall. The analysis would compare the content of the diet in the cases and controls, controlling for possible confounding variables.

In a cohort study, detailed data on diet are collected in a large group of people free of bowel disease; the cohort is followed up for several years and all new cases of bowel cancer are identified. The risk of disease is then related to the fat content of the diet at the beginning and during the study. This study design presents many logistic problems but systematic bias is less of a problem.

3.3 Random error is the variation of an observed value from the true population value due to chance alone. It can be reduced by increasing the size of the study sample and improving the reliability of the measurement method.

3.4 Systematic error occurs when there is a tendency to produce results that differ systematically from the true values. The main sources of systematic error are selection bias and measurement bias.

Selection bias occurs when the people who take part in a study are systematically different from those who do not. The possibility of selection bias can be reduced by a clear and explicit definition of the criteria for entry into the study, a knowledge of the natural history and management of the disease, and a high response rate.

Measurement bias occurs when there is a systematic error in measurement or classification of the participants in a study. It can be reduced by good study design, involving, for example, standard criteria for the disease, detailed attention to the quality control of measurement methods, and the collection of data without knowledge of the disease status of the participant.

3.5 Relative risk (RR) is used in prospective studies (e.g. cohort) while Odds Ratio (OR) is calculated in a case-control (retrospective) study. In a case-control study, there are those who have the disease and those who do not (including those who are exposed and those who are not). It is therefore of interest to calculate the ratio of the probability of occurrence of an event to that of non occurrence, that is to determine the chances of those not sick becoming sick.

A relative risk is almost never calculated in case-control studies. In calculating a RR, one is comparing the incidence of those exposed and incidence of those not exposed (probability of occurrence of a disease in the exposed and in the non-exposed).

3.6 In the case of a rare disease (for example, most cancers), RR and OR are very similar. This is because the odds ratio formula is: sick exposed x non-sick not exposed / sick not exposed x non-sick exposed.

3.7 Maternal age is a confounder: it is correlated with birth order and is a risk factor even if birth order is low. In another sample where all mothers are below 30 years, no association with birth order would be found.

Birth Order ⟶ Down's Syndrome

Maternal age

One way to avoid confounding would be to stratify by maternal age.

Chapter 4

4.1   The sum of the n = 10 observations is 679.1 kg; the mean is 67.91; the median is 67.3—note that there are two observations with values of 67.3 that are in the middle of the group after they have been put into order; the variance is 104.03 kg^2; the standard deviation is 10.20 kg; and the standard error is 3.23 kg.

4.2   The median is often used to report personal income for a group since it is much less affected by a few very high income levels, which can sometimes make the average income for the group much higher than the levels for most of the members.

4.3   There are two major differences among these models. First, while the independent variables can be the same for all three, the dependent variables are quite different, with the dependent variable for linear regression being a continuous variable, for logistic regression being a representation for a dichotomous variable such as the presence or absence of some characteristic, and for survival models being the measure of a time interval from some specified point until a pre-specified event occurs. Coefficients for linear regression represent either differences between means or slopes, for logistic regression represent odds ratios and for survival models represent hazard rate ratios.

4.4   The narrower the better. This is true since the confidence interval concept is such that, for example, the sample mean, which is an estimate of the mean for the population from which the sample was taken, is in the middle of the confidence interval. Further, one would expect 95% of such intervals to contain the true value of the population mean and the shorter the interval the closer the sample mean is likely to be to the population mean.

4.5   In general, tables presenting data or results should "stand alone" in a manuscript or report. This means that the reader should be able to interpret the data presented without reference to the text or to other documents. The table title is essential for this purpose. Data tables typically are made up of a set of cells and the table title should state "what, how classified, where and when" in reference to the information in the cells. An example is "Number and percent of participants, classified by age, race and gender, CARDIA Study, 2006.

4.6   For this situation, $b_1 = \text{mean}_{males} - \text{mean}_{females} = 5.0$ kg, adjusted for the other independent variables in the model.

4.7   For this situation, $b_1 = 0.5$ represents the slope for the relationship between age and body weight. It is interpreted as the increment in body weight per one year increment in age, which, in this case, means that body weight increases 0.5 kg per year of increase in age.

Chapter 5

5.1   The process of determining whether an observed association is likely to be causal.

5.2   This means that some causal factors lead to exposures to other factors that are the direct cause of the disease. For instance, low income is associated with a low intake of fruit and vegetables in the United Kingdom (Figure 5.9). Low intake of fruit and vegetables is in turn associated with a higher diastolic blood pressure. Income determines diet, which determines a health outcome; a hierarchy of causes.

5.3   Attributable fraction for smoking = (602–58)/602 = 0.904, or 90%. Attributable fraction for asbestos exposure = (602–123)/602 = 0.796, or 80%. Eliminating one of the factors can reduce the incidence of lung cancer to the extent indicated by these substantial fractions. Decisions about prevention programs will depend also on the likelihood of success in reducing exposures to either factor. Reducing smoking habits among asbestos workers is obviously important, but if asbestos exposure can be completely eliminated by technology changes, this could actually achieve even more prevention. In order to calculate population attributable risks it is necessary also to know what proportion of the population is smoking and what proportion is exposed to asbestos at work.

5.4   The criteria include: the temporal nature of the relation, plausibility, consistency, the strength of the association, the dose-response relationship, reversibility, and the study design. Of these criteria, only temporality is essential; ultimately, judgment is required.

5.5   On the basis of this evidence alone one could not be certain that the association was causal; a policy of withdrawing the drug could not, therefore, be recommended. The effects of bias (measurement, selection) and confounding in the study and the role of chance would need to be assessed. If bias and chance are unlikely to be the explanation, then the causal criteria can be applied. In fact, when all the evidence was considered in such a study in New Zealand, the investigators concluded that the association was likely to be causal.[28]

5.6   A temporal relationship is most important. Did the patients consume the oil before or after they fell ill? If there is no information on the chemical in the oil that is associated with the disease, it is impossible to assess plausibility or consistency. Therefore strength and dose-response relationship based on information on oil consumption could be the next matters for study. As it is urgent priority to find the likely cause, the most suitable approach would be to conduct a case-control study, together with chemical analysis of the oil and of biological monitoring samples. It would be prudent to intervene as soon as a temporal relationship has been clearly established and the strength of association appears great, particularly if there is no other likely cause.

5.7   It is acceptable for acute effects that occur within hours or days of the exposure. It is using the exposed group as its own control. On hot days the population is exposed and on cooler days the same population serves as a control. If daily data are used, it is considered that the population size or character does not change during the study period and confounding should be limited.

5.8 Meta-analysis combines data from more than one study in order to achieve more stable and precise conclusions concerning causal associations. To use this method each study needs to have used the same exposure and health outcome variables and the basic population characteristics (age, sex, etc.) should also be the same in each study.

5.9 The risk of ischaemic heart disease is about twice as high in the lower fruit and vegetable consumption quintile as in the upper quintile (Figure 5.8). The fruit and vegetable intake levels in Figure 5.9 for the highest and lowest quintiles are approximately 300 and 150 grams per day, respectively. Combining these estimates indicates that lower income groups may have four times higher ischaemic heart disease risk in relation to fruit and vegetable consumption than the higher income groups. Clearly, public health actions and policies need to find ways to make fruit and vegetable intake more common in low income households. Figure 5.9 indicates that at least in the United Kingdom food prices may be a key factor. Just like taxes are applied to unhealthy products, such as tobacco, it may be worth providing subsidies for fruit and vegetable production and distribution. School lunches can also be a target for improved diets in this respect.

Chapter 6

6.1   The four levels of prevention are: primordial, primary, secondary and tertiary. A comprehensive programme for the prevention of stroke would include activities at each of these levels.

Primordial prevention would involve stopping the rise of population levels of the major risk factors for common chronic diseases including stroke.

Primary prevention includes both population prevention through public health legislation and environmental changes addressed at the whole population, as well as a "high risk" strategy targeting treatment at individuals at high overall risk of an acute stroke event.

Secondary prevention programmes would involve the early treatment and rehabilitation. If people who have already had a heart attack or stroke are included in the high risk prevention strategy, in effect, this merges the high risk strategy with secondary prevention.

Tertiary prevention involves rehabilitation of patients suffering from the long-term effects or sequelae of stroke.

6.2   This cannot be answered in general terms. Each potential prevention programme needs to be assessed in context. Each programme must be balanced by an appropriate mix of population and high-risk activities based on a number of factors including the levels of diabetes and obesity, the major risk factors, the affordability of clinical care, and issues of equity. The challenge is not to choose between one or the other approach, but to move investment towards populations approaches while improving the quality of the high-risk approaches that are in operation.

6.3   For a disease to be suitable for screening it must be serious, the natural history of the disease must be understood, there should be a long period between development of the first signs and appearance of overt disease, an effective treatment must be available and, usually, the prevalence of the disease must be high.

6.4   All study designs have been used to evaluate screening programmes. Randomized controlled trials are ideal, but cross-sectional, cohort and case-control studies are also used.

Chapter 7

7.1   The proportion of deaths due to infectious diseases has declined in the USA since 1950 and chronic diseases have become more important. Demographic change, with an increased proportion of elderly people, is one explanation. It would be helpful to have age-specific mortality data for individual diseases to allow further examination of the trends. Two general explanations for a decrease in age-specific infectious disease mortality have been advanced. First, there has been a general reduction in host susceptibility through improved nutrition and sanitation. This is likely to be the most important factor, particularly in respect of the early improvement. Secondly, specific medical interventions may have played a part, particularly since the 1950s.

7.2   A record of weekly (or daily) cases of measles found by clinics and health practitioners in the district should be kept. The "normal" background level (perhaps two cases or fewer per week) and a threshold level for an incipient epidemic (perhaps twice or three times the background level) should be established. When the threshold is exceeded, preventive action should be taken.

7.3   The chain of infection for foodborne salmonella goes from faecal material (either from humans or animals, particularly chickens) to water or food which, when consumed, leads to infection. Alternatively, it goes from faecal material to hands and then to food (during food preparation), which again leads to infection.

7.4   The revised International Health Regulations (2005) establishes a single code of procedures and practices for routine public health measures.
The IHR (2005) does not include an enforcement mechanism for the countries which fail to comply with its provisions.
Countries will need to meet the human and financial requirements for

- developing, strengthening and maintaining the necessary public health capacities, and mobilizing the resources necessary for that purpose;
- adopting the necessary legal and administrative provisions
- designating a national IHR Focal Point
  assessment and notification of events occurring within their territory that may constitute a public health emergency of international concern, and;
- implementing measures at certain international airports, ports and ground crossings, including routine inspection and control activities.

7.5   The four levels of prevention are: primordial, primary, secondary and tertiary. A comprehensive programme for the prevention of tuberculosis would include activities at each of these levels.
Primordial prevention can involve preventing the entry of infectious cases into a healthy population. People from endemic areas can be required to provide evidence that they are not infected before entering non-endemic areas. In addition, the factors that increase the risk of tuberculosis, such as overcrowding, poverty and poor nutrition can be addressed.
Primary prevention includes immunization and case-finding, to avoid spread of the disease.

Secondary prevention programmes involve the early and effective treatment of infected people.

Tertiary prevention involves rehabilitation of patients suffering from the long-term effects or sequelae of tuberculosis and its treatment.

Chapter 8

8.1 The term is strictly a contradiction in that epidemiology deals with populations whereas clinical medicine deals with individual patients. However, it is appropriate because clinical epidemiology studies populations of patients.

8.2 The limitation of this definition is that there are no biological grounds for using an arbitrary cut-off point as the basis for distinguishing normal from abnormal. For many diseases the risk increases with increasing levels of risk factors and much of the burden of disease falls on people in the normal range.

8.3 The sensitivity of the new test=8/10×100=80%; its specificity= 9000/10000×100=90%. The new test appears good; a decision on whether to use it in the general population requires information on its positive predictive value, which in this case is 8/1008=0.008. This very low value is related to the low prevalence of the disease. For this reason, it would not be appropriate to recommend general use of the test.

8.4 The positive predictive value of a screening test is the proportion of the people with positive results who actually have the disease. The major determinant of the positive predictive value is the prevalence of the pre-clinical disease in the screened population. If the population is at low risk for the disease, most of the positive results will be false. Predictive value also depends on the sensitivity and specificity of the test.

8.5 Advantages of randomized controlled trials are that they allow a calculation of:

- the benefit of a treatment relative to those who did not receive the treatment - or the relative risk reduction (RRR)
- the actual benefit of a treatment (or risk of the event without the therapy). This is expressed as the difference in the rates between the two groups - the absolute risk reduction (ARR)
- the number needed to treat (NNT) to prevent one event over a given period of time.

8.6 a) 2.65%
b) 2.35%
c) 12%
d) 0.30% (2.65%-2.35%)
e) The NNT to prevent 1 CVD event over 6.4 years is 333 (1 / =.30%)
f) 2,100 (6.4 years x 333)
g) 3 CVD events prevented per 1000 women.

8.7 Some of the potential problems with this metaanalysis include the following:

- Aspirin dose, duration of treatment, and lengths of follow up were unlikely to be uniform in the 6 selected studies.
- Even with pooling six large trials, the numbers of individual outcome events were infrequent because of the low risk of the populations studied, thus reducing the power of the study to detect differences.
- Only analysis of data from participants from all the available trials would have allowed an examination of aspirin benefit in particular subgroups who may have benefited.

- Meta-analysis is retrospective research, subject to the methodological deficiencies of each included study.

8.8 On the basis of this study, it could be concluded that low-dose aspirin is associated with a reduction on cardiovascular events in both men and women but also associated with a significant risk of major bleeding. Recommendations would include the need to explain to a patient both the beneficial and harmful effects of aspirin before considering aspirin for the primary prevention of cardiovascular disease in low risk patients. This information should be conveyed in a clinically significant way - in terms of number-needed-to-treat (and number-needed-to-harm) or absolute risk reduction rather than relative risk reduction.

Chapter 9

9.1 (a) Children, as they develop the effects at lower blood levels.

(b) Changes in neurobehavioural function, as these develop at lower blood levels.

9.2 (a) An increasing relative risk of lung cancer.

(b) Because it is known that the total amount (dose) of asbestos particles (fibres) inhaled (concentration×duration of exposure) is what determines the risk of asbestos-induced disease.

9.3 The answer will depend on the toxic substance chosen. The types of biological materials to consider are: blood, urine, hair, saliva, nail clippings, faeces, and possibly biopsy materials.

9.4 You should start by collecting case histories, holding discussions with local medical services and making visits to suspected industries in order to develop the hypothesis for study. Then a case-control study of lung cancer within the city should be done.

9.5 Information on deaths in previous years (without smog) and on the age-specific causes of death would be helpful. Evidence from animal experiments might serve to document the effects of the smog (in fact, the live animals on display at London's Smithfield Meat Market also suffered). The close time association of the smog and its pollutants with an increase in deaths is strong evidence for a causal relationship.

9.6 The healthy worker effect refers to the low background morbidity and mortality rates that are found in both exposed and unexposed groups in the workplace. The reason is that, in order to be active in an occupation, people need to be reasonably healthy. Ill and disabled people are selectively excluded from the study groups. If a control group is chosen from the general population, bias may be introduced because the group is inherently less healthy.

9.7 Situations where: a. well defined geographic sub-area definitions and census or other population data exist; b. the exposure of interest can be measured or modeled in the same geographic sub-areas; c. data on exposures and effects for each geographic sub-area can be assembled for appropriate time periods.

9.8 Driving cars or motor cycles: seat belts, speed limits, alcohol limits, crash helmets. Housing and workplace design. Safety features of household products, e.g. electrical products, child safety lids on jars and medicine containers. Life jackets in boats, etc.

Chapter 10

10.1 Using the guiding principles of the Bangkok Charter towards the development of healthy public policy would include such actions as:

- Advocate: advocacy is required to ensure governments fulfil all the obligations of the Framework Convention on Tobacco Control to prevent tobacco use in children.
- Invest: the resources to address the underlying determinants of tobacco use in children e.g., deprivation, poverty and alienation.
- Build capacity: ensure there is sufficient human capacity to deliver the programmes, and sufficient financial resources.
- Regulate and legislate: children should be protected from the advertising and promotion of all tobacco products.
- Build alliances: government and civil society should join forces to implement the required actions.

10.2 Various questions must be asked at different stages of the planning cycle:

Assessing the burden

- How common are falls in the elderly?
- What epidemiological data are available?
- What studies are required?

Identifying the causes

- How can falls be prevented?
- Monitoring activities and measuring progress (e.g. indicators)

Effective interventions

- What treatment resources are available?

Determining efficiency

- How effective are the treatment services?
- What rehabilitation services are available and are they effective?
- How does the cost of these services compare with their effectiveness?

Implementing interventions

- Should new types of services be established and tested?

Evaluation

- Has the occurrence of falls changed since the new services were provided?

10.3 In developing a national policy, the following parameters need to be considered:

- Burden: are noncommunicable diseases a priority issue in terms of mortality and morbidity? How reliable are the national data? What are the priority noncommunicable diseases?
- Causation: is there local evidence on the causal importance of the common risk factors? Is such evidence needed?
- Effectiveness: is there local evidence on the effectiveness and cost effectiveness of standard noncommunicable disease interventions; both at population and individual levels?
- Efficiency: is a noncommunicable disease policy the best use of existing resources?
- Implementation: what are the implementation priorities for both populations and individuals?
- Monitoring and measuring progress: is there a monitoring and evaluation plan in place? What are the priorities for evaluation?

Chapter 11

11.1 This was a well-designed and well-conducted randomized controlled trial on the use of aspirin in the primary prevention of cardiovascular mortality. The study was conducted on male American physicians who, it turned out, were very healthy. Out of a total of 261 000 physicians, 22 000 took part. The healthy state of the physicians meant that the study had less statistical power than originally planned. Extrapolating the results to other populations is difficult because of the exclusions that limited the study population to physicians likely to comply and not to have adverse side-effects. These design features increased the likelihood of a high success rate. Confirmation of the benefits of aspirin is required from other studies. It is always necessary to balance benefits against risks (gastrointestinal side-effects, increased risk of bleeding, etc.).

11.2 Ecological evidence on asthma therapy is related to a suggested increase in asthma mortality. It would be difficult to agree with the conclusion. Information is presented only on people dying with asthma; no information is provided on asthmatics not dying. This study is a case series; there are no controls. Such a study, however, points to the desirability of further investigation. In this case a more formal examination of asthma mortality trends has identified a new epidemic of asthma deaths, the cause of which is still under investigation, although a particular drug has apparently contributed substantially to it.

Index